HAPTICS FOR TELEOPERATED SURGICAL ROBOTIC SYSTEMS

T0324512

New Frontiers in Robotics — 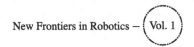 Vol. 1

HAPTICS FOR TELEOPERATED SURGICAL ROBOTIC SYSTEMS

M Tavakoli
Harvard University, USA

R V Patel
University of Western Ontario, Canada

M Moallem
Simon Fraser University, Canada

A Aziminejad
University of Western Ontario, Canada

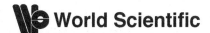 **World Scientific**

NEW JERSEY · LONDON · SINGAPORE · BEIJING · SHANGHAI · HONG KONG · TAIPEI · CHENNAI

Published by

World Scientific Publishing Co. Pte. Ltd.

5 Toh Tuck Link, Singapore 596224

USA office: 27 Warren Street, Suite 401-402, Hackensack, NJ 07601

UK office: 57 Shelton Street, Covent Garden, London WC2H 9HE

British Library Cataloguing-in-Publication Data
A catalogue record for this book is available from the British Library.

HAPTICS FOR TELEOPERATED SURGICAL ROBOTIC SYSTEMS
New Frontiers in Robotics — Vol. 1

ISBN-13 978-981-281-315-2
ISBN-10 981-281-315-2

Printed in Singapore.

To our families

Preface

Surgery traditionally involves making a large incision to access the part of a patient's body that requires attention. This approach is referred to as open surgery. Minimally invasive surgery (MIS), also called endoscopic surgery, is an alternative to open surgery in which an endoscope (camera) and long instruments are inserted into the body cavity through small incisions about 1 cm across. Instead of looking directly at the area being treated, the physician monitors the procedure via the endoscope.

Because of the small incision size, MIS significantly reduces trauma to the body, post-operative pain and length of hospital stay compared to open surgery. It may potentially benefit the health care system through cost savings as well. For example, traditional gallbladder surgery requires a six-day hospital stay and up to six weeks for a full recovery and leaves a six-inch scar. However, if operated in a minimally invasive mode, gallbladder patients usually leave the hospital the same or the next day and are fully recovered after a week with the scar barely visible after a few months. Apart from societal benefits from faster recovery, this leads to savings on pain medications, nursing care and overhead costs in an expensive clinical setting.

Despite these benefits, endoscopic surgery has some drawbacks such as lack of dexterity and manipulation capability for the surgeon. Such problems can be overcome by using robots to assist surgeons during interventions. A surgical robot (slave) in conjunction with a computer controlled surgeon-robot interface (master), where a surgeon sits and performs the procedure while watching the surgical field via a 2-D or 3-D imaging system, can also make the surgeon less fatigued and the operations much more precise. A major deficiency of the current master-slave robotic systems for surgery is the lack of the sensation of touch, or haptic perception, for the surgeon. Haptic feedback has the potential to provide superior performance and reliability in master-slave robot-assisted interventions.

Motivated by this application, we have been investigating various issues associated with incorporating haptics in robot-assisted MIS. The results of the research are summarized in this monograph. A number of the key results are applicable to haptics-based teleoperated systems in general. The following is an outline of each chapter of the monograph and how the chapters relate to each other:

Chapter 1 starts by describing interventions that can take advantage of the benefits offered by robotics. Next, a classification of robotic tools and manipulators, which may be used in various types of surgery or therapy is provided. Then, to lay the ground for studying haptic interaction in robot-assisted interventions, some of the available haptic devices and the previous research on haptic surgical teleoperation are surveyed.

While Chapter 1 provides a broad overview of the types of surgeries and therapies that can benefit from robotics, the types of robots that can assist surgeons, and haptic interaction during robot-assisted surgery and therapy, Chapters 2 and 3 focus on a specific intervention (MIS) and a specific class of robotic systems (master-slave teleoperation systems) with the objective of incorporating haptic feedback. Studies in Chapters 4, 5, 6 and 7 are also done in the context of that specific intervention although they are not necessarily limited to it.

Chapters 2 to 7 deal with devices and methods required for incorporating haptic interaction in *master-slave robotic systems* for *minimally invasive endoscopic interventions*. In terms of devices, incorporating haptic feedback into a robotic MIS system calls for a surgical end-effector that can measure its interaction with tissue in the form of forces or torques, as well as a force-reflective user interface. Chapters 2 and 3 discuss the design of two such devices for an endoscopic surgery environment.

In Chapter 2, a novel robotic end-effector is described that meets the requirements of endoscopic surgery and is sensorized for force/torque feedback. The endoscopic end-effector is capable of non-invasively measuring its interaction with tissue in all degrees of freedom available during endoscopic manipulation. It is also capable of remotely actuating a tip and measuring its interaction with the environment without using any sensors on the jaws. The sensorized end-effector can be used as the last arm of a surgical robot to incorporate haptic feedback.

Chapter 3 discusses the design of a user interface that is capable of providing force feedback in all the degrees of freedom available during endoscopic surgery. Using the Jacobian matrix of the haptic interface and its singular values, methods are proposed for the analysis and optimization of the interface performance with regard to the accuracy of force feedback, the range of applicable forces, and the accuracy of control.

It has been shown that fixed impedance-reflecting controllers cannot preserve master-slave position tracking when the environment impedance changes. In Chapter 4, a neural network is used to implement adaptive inverse dynamics control of a PHANToM haptic device, which is commonly used in haptics-based master-slave teleoperation research. Experimental results show that the neural network controller successfully represents the inverse dynamics of the PHANToM and can adapt to changes in the dynamics to maintain master-slave tracking.

In Chapter 5, the force-reflective user interface of Chapter 3 is used with the sensorized surgical instrument of Chapter 2 to form a master-slave testbed for studying haptic interaction in an endoscopic surgery environment. For experiments involving a single degree-of-freedom surgical task on soft tissue (palpation), first the dynamics of the master and the slave including friction effects are modeled and the model parameters are identified (Appendix D). Since the master is not equipped with a force/torque sensor, a state observer based on the identified dynamical model of the master is utilized to estimate the force exerted by the operator's hand. In this chapter, the added benefits of using force sensors that measure hand/master and slave/environment interactions and utilizing local feedback loops on teleoperation transparency are investigated. We compare two-channel and the four-channel bilateral control systems in terms of stability and transparency, and study the stability and performance robustness of the four-channel method against non-idealities arisen during bilateral control implementation including master-slave communication latency and changes in the environment dynamics.

As mentioned before, providing a surgeon with information regarding contacts made between instruments and tissue during robot-assisted interventions can improve task efficiency and reliability. However, it has been established that due to major difficulties in design and technology, incorporating full haptic interaction in today's complex surgical systems demands fundamental system re-designs and upgrades as well as long-term financial and R & D commitments from the manufacturers. Therefore, in the short term and for some applications involving robotic surgery, it may be more cost-effective and advantageous to provide substitute modes of sensory feedback to the surgeon. In Chapter 6, alternative methods for feedback of such information to the surgeon are discussed. It is hypothesized that various modalities of contact feedback have the potential to enhance performance in a robot-assisted minimally invasive environment. To verify the hypothesis, the master-slave test-bed is used to compare users' performance in doing a single degree-of-freedom surgical task (lump localization) for different modalities of contact feedback. In this chapter, it is also studied whether haptic feedback or substitution for haptic feedback can help improve task performance under degraded visual conditions.

In master-slave telesurgery, the time delay experienced in the communication between the master and the slave can cause instability in the teleoperated system. A wave-based control architecture can theoretically make a bilateral teleoperation system insensitive to communication time delays through encoding velocity and force information prior to transmission. However, transparency of the teleoperation system is altered by this process. In Chapter 7, we propose two different approaches for improving transparency of a wave-based delay-compensated teleoperation system: direct force reflection in a two-channel control architecture, which uses the same number of channels as the traditional position error-based control scheme with wave variables and, four-channel wave-based control architecture, which is capable of achieving ideal transparency in the presence of time delays. In order to present a comprehensive performance comparison, we quantify the transparency of each approach through experiments on the master-slave system described earlier.

This monograph is primarily aimed at the medical robotics and haptics communities. Due to its practical nature, it will be of use to a wide range of readers with interests and background in robotics, teleoperation, haptics, virtual reality, sensor technology, human-machine interaction, and minimally invasive surgery and therapy.

The funding for the research described in this monograph was provided by the Natural Sciences and Engineering Research Council (NSERC) of Canada under grants RGPIN-1345 and RGPIN- 227612, the Ontario Research and Development Challenge Fund under grant 00-May-0709 and infrastructure grants from the Canada Foundation for Innovation awarded to the London Health Sciences Centre (CSTAR) and the University of Western Ontario. This support is gratefully acknowledged.

Contents

List of Figures

List of Tables

Chapter 1

Introduction

Robotics technology has recently found extensive use in surgical and therapeutic procedures. The purpose of this chapter is to give an overview of the robotic tools which may be used in various types of surgery or therapy. The chapter starts with a general classification of interventions that can take advantage of the benefits offered by robots. Next, the literature is surveyed regarding robotic tools and manipulators for applications in surgery and therapy. Both the current commercial components and those components still under development are reported. Finally, to lay the groundwork for studying haptic interaction in robot-assisted surgery and therapy, some of the available haptic devices and previous research on haptic surgical teleoperation are surveyed.

1.1 Robot-Assisted Intervention: Benefits and Applications

Using robots in medical interventions can offer benefits including high accuracy, fine manipulation capability, good repeatability, high reliability, lack of fatigue, etc. The use of robots can also benefit the patients through reducing morbidity, traumas, errors and operation times.

Most of the interventions that can take advantage of the above benefits are either accurate procedures or interventions involving minimal access to the body organ that needs attention. Accurate procedures can either be on a scale uncomfortable for an unaided hand (e.g., eye surgery or microsurgery [63]) or can require high geometric accuracy (e.g., orthopedic surgery [66]). Another example of accurate procedures requiring "super-human" precision is neurosurgery where tissue damage must strictly be avoided [81]. Minimal access procedures are procedures performed through incisions made into the patient's body (e.g., cardiac surgery [78] or urologic surgery [128, 50]), interventions performed through natural orifices in the human body (e.g., through the gastrointestinal tract [111]), intravascular interventions (e.g., intravascular neurosurgery [98]), etc. While minimally invasive surgery makes procedures less traumatic, the precision, dexterity and reliability of surgical maneuvers can be considerably enhanced by the use of robots.

1.2   Robotics Technology for Surgery and Therapy

Devices and systems for surgery and therapy can either be directly used by a surgeon to perform an intervention (augmenting devices) or can perform secondary functions to support the surgeon (supporting devices) [135]. Each of these types can be classified into different groups, as discussed next.

1.2.1   *Augmenting devices and systems*

As the name implies, an augmenting device extends the surgeon's ability in performing an operation. Depending on their modes of interaction with the surgeon, robotic devices or systems can be categorized into the following groups:

1.2.1.1   *Hand-held tools*

One advantage of using hand-held tools is that they do not constrain the surgeon and involve minimal changes to the operating room. The down side is that with purely hand-held instruments, a robot cannot be used to physically support heavier instruments. Also without any robotic arms, instruments cannot be locked in position and precisely controlled maneuvers (e.g. as required during microsurgery) are not possible [135]. The hand-held devices are mostly sensorized and can be divided into several categories as follows depending on their functionalities:

Master-slave combined instruments   Unlike master-slave *telemanipulators*, a master-slave combined instrument comprises of a master interface and a slave tool that are combined through the instrument body and enable the surgeon to operate the instrument near the patient together with other conventional surgical tools. Master-slave combined instruments can be used to enhance the surgeon's situational awareness and/or capabilities during surgery. A master-slave combined instrument for suturing and ligaturing tasks during general surgery is discussed in [90]. The surgeon is responsible for large and quick motions of the instrument while the master handle embedded in this instrument directs the fine motion of the tip.

The idea of master-slave combined teleoperation can also be applied to enhance manipulation of tissue by enabling the surgeon to better sense the instrument's interaction with tissue. The tool described in [25] has a steerable tip with sensors for detecting the tip's interaction with the tissue. This device can be used as a hand-held tool for traditional arthroscopy or as part of a system for computer-assisted arthroscopy. The device has a semi-automatic collision avoidance feature for preventing contact between the tip and some pre-selected environments.

Instruments for reducing hand tremors Hand tremors can be critical in delicate procedures such as ophthalmological and neurological surgery especially when the surgeon becomes fatigued. A totally hand-held instrument for tremor reduction in microsurgery is discussed in [4]. In this device, hand motions are first detected by sensors. Next, a frequency-domain algorithm is used to identify the tremors from the desired motions of the hand. Then, the tremors are compensated for by piezoelectric actuators embedded in the manipulator system of the hand-held device.

Instruments for increased dexterity and navigation capability During intravascular interventions and interventions through natural orifices, long and slender catheters are used for diagnosis purposes or treating abnormalities. In intravascular neurosurgery, for example, a micro-catheter is advanced through vessels toward the brain while the surgeon monitors the location of the catheter using an X-ray display. When the tip of the micro-catheter reaches the targeted site, various substances or drugs can be delivered or a narrowed portion of the blood vessel can be opened up by inflating a micro-balloon attached to the tip [98]. However, due to the lack of dexterity of present micro-catheters, guiding them through complex vessels and branches is a difficult task for the surgeon.

To develop highly dexterous intravascular catheters, continuous flexible stems that can be bent using smart actuators may be used. Fukuda et al. [37] discuss a shape memory alloy (SMA) based micro-catheter with two degrees of freedom. Haga et al. [47] discuss an active micro-catheter actuated by distributed SMA coils and equipped with a miniature ultrasonic transducer to perform intraureteral ultrasonography of kidney. Electrostrictive polymer actuators are also proving to be another possible alternative for

controlled bending of catheters [118, 75]. Narumiya proposes the integration of sensors at the tip of a micro-catheter to inform the surgeon about
the interactions occurring between the catheter and the blood vessels for
optimizing the micro-catheter's travel path with least resistance (i.e. least
trauma to the patient) [97].

Instruments for measurement purposes   Hand-held tools can be sensorized and used for measuring the mechanical properties of tissues. The
experimental data collected from the sensors can help to find tissue models
for surgical simulators both in terms of deformations and force reflections.
A sensor-equipped grasper for in-vivo detection of tissue force-deformation
properties is discussed in [12]. Similarly, indentors or tissue stretchers have
been developed for this purpose [108].

Sensorized hand-held devices can also be used for defining and assessing
desirable surgical performance by measuring interactions occurring between
the surgeon and a tool [114], or between a tool and tissue [95]. The data
obtained from the sensors can be used for objective surgical skills evaluation
[113], and for surgical robot design.

1.2.1.2   *Cooperatively-controlled tools*

In cooperative manipulation, the surgeon and the robot both hold the surgical device – the surgeon provides control and the robot provides precision,
sensitivity and guidance. Such devices act as guidance systems with which
the surgeon's motions are constrained. Cooperatively-controlled devices
can be active (force controlled) or passive mechanisms as discussed next.

Force controlled devices   Force-controlled cooperatively-controlled
robots try to minimize the forces exerted on the robot's end-effector through
complying with the surgeon's hand movements. For example, in the Steady-
Hand robot [134], force sensors measure the force exerted by the surgeon
on the tool and by the tool on the tissue. Using these measurements, the
Steady-Hand slows the surgeon's motion and mechanically filters tremor.
This system is being evaluated for microsurgical tasks in ophthalmology
and otology [116, 76].

Another example of force-controlled cooperatively-controlled robots is
the ROBODOC system [137] for joint replacement surgery. When the patient's bones are ready to receive the implant, the patient's bones are fix-
ated to the robot's base. Since the robot is force controlled, the surgeon's
hand can guide it to an initial position. After this cooperative manipula-

tion phase, the robot cuts the desired shape according to the pre-operative plans while monitoring cutting forces, bone motion, etc. The cooperative mode of operation seems to be popular with surgeons because they become more involved and remain more in control during the procedure. The ROBODOC system has been used during primary and revision total hip replacement surgery [13], and knee surgery [149].

The cooperative control mode has been also incorporated into the LARS system [136], the Neurobot system [125], and the ACROBOT system [67]. While ROBODOC was cooperatively controlled during the initial positioning only, some of the other systems have been used for cooperative control during the intervention itself.

Passive devices A passive guidance mechanism that is held cooperatively by the robot and the surgeon and constrains the possible actions of the surgeon to what is authorized in the planning is described in [119].

1.2.1.3 *Teleoperated tools*

In Teleoperated (or master-slave) surgery, the movements of a surgical robot (slave) are controlled via a surgeon's console (master). Master-slave robotic operations can solve many of the problems encountered in conventional surgery in terms of ergonomics, dexterity, fine manipulation capability, and haptic feedback capability for the surgeon.

The most prominent commercial surgical robotic systems are the da Vinci and the Zeus systems [8]. The latter is no longer available. In these dual-handed systems, two slave robots manipulate the surgical instruments and another slave robot controls the camera (see Figure 1.1). In the da Vinci, a fourth arm is also available. With these systems, the surgeon becomes less fatigued sitting at a comfortable and ergonomic console. The end-effector of the da Vinci robot includes a wrist that adds three rotations and one tool tip actuation (i.e. pitch, yaw, roll, and gripping at the wrist) to the degrees of freedom. The Zeus wrist adds one rotation. Both the da Vinci and the Zeus systems allow precise movements through scaling the hand motions (up to a factor of 5:1 for the da Vinci and 10:1 for the Zeus), and filter out hand tremors. These systems eliminate the motion reversal experienced with conventional endoscopic tools (chop-stick effect), yet do not presently provide feedback of tactile/force (haptic) sensations to the surgeon.

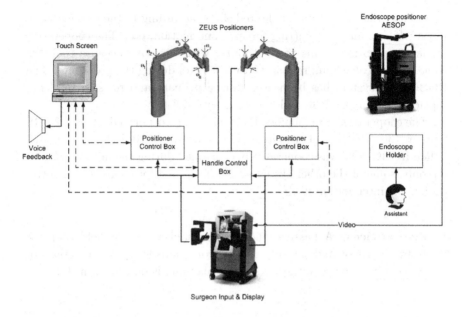

Fig. 1.1   A block diagram of the Zeus system from Intuitive Surgical, Inc.

Sensorized tools for incorporating haptic interaction   A miniature tactile sensor array has been mounted at the tip of a laparoscopic tool [45]. This sensor consists of an array of capacitive sensor cells whose capacitance will changes in response to pressure, thus detecting any contact with the environment. A similar example is a tactile sensor array mounted on the jaw of a grasping tool [60]. In this example, signals from the sensor are transmitted to a tactile display so that surgeons can sense pressure distribution on the instruments for localization of arteries and tumors.

An actuated and sensor-equipped grasper capable of grasping force control and position sensing is reported in [115]. This tool is used with an actuated and sensor-equipped finger loop interface capable of providing force feedback to the surgeon. A laparoscopic grasper that can measure interactions with tissues in three degrees of freedom is reported in [142].

Tools for increased dexterity in teleoperation   Articulation can be used to provide rotational movement at the distal end of a robotic end-effector using one joint. Compared to multi-joint articulation, the advantages of single-joint design include relative simplicity and low space requirements for movement inside the body. The disadvantages are that the joint does not leave much room for other linkages to pass through and has a very sharp bending angle [33].

An articulated robotic end-effector (together with a haptic-enabled user interface) for laparoscopic surgery is reported in [20]. The dexterous manipulator allows complex surgical operations to be performed.

1.2.1.4 *Autonomous tools*

Autonomous instruments A robotic system that can perform certain tasks autonomously can reduce the strain on the surgeon and shorten the operation time. A robotic end-effector for autonomous suturing and knot tying is discussed in [69].

Autonomous systems Surgeons are more interested in assist tools with a degree of intelligence and reaction capability than in full-fledged systems that automate the surgeons' role by using imaging and robotics technology. The Minerva system for neurosurgery is an example of the technological opportunities and the clinical dismay [26]. However, there is interest in developing autonomous robotic systems for biopsy (e.g. PAKY-RCM [23]), orthopedic surgery (e.g. ROBODOC [137], Arthrobot [77]), neurosurgery (e.g. NeuroMate [65]), etc.

1.2.2 *Supporting devices and systems*

Unlike augmenting devices which are directly used by surgeons to perform interventions, supporting devices perform secondary functions such as holding endoscopes or surgical instruments. It is desirable to improve these systems so that they become more independent of the surgeon and operate with more autonomy.

1.2.2.1 *Positioning/stabilization purposes*

Positioning stands for tools A positioning stand can help the surgeon to position and lock endoscopic tools without the need for an assistant surgeon. The optimal design of the kinematic configuration of such a positioning stand is discussed in [31].

Camera positioners/stabilizers In conventional endoscopic surgery, an assistant holds and manipulates the endoscope through commands from the surgeon. In this mode, the camera may not be positioned accurately or timely enough mainly due to the fatigue and hand tremors of the assistant.

Instead, a robotic manipulator can be used for endoscopic camera manipulation as reported in [103]. In these systems, the surgeon's command can be issued through a joystick, foot pedals, voice, head movements, facial expressions, etc. Alternatively, surgical instruments can be visually tracked [43], thus providing the information on the desired position of the endoscope to the positioner robot's control loop [154].

Ultrasound probe positioner   More recently, there has been interest in robotic systems for manipulating ultrasound probes [92, 1] . Most of this activity has targeted diagnostic procedures. However, these systems can potentially be used, for example, during precise ultrasound-guided biopsies and other interventional procedures.

Stabilizers for surgeon's hand   A moving support for the surgeon's hand that can track the heart motions, thus allowing for coronary artery bypass grafting (CABG) surgery on the beating heart, is discussed in [144].

1.2.2.2   *Increasing device dexterity or autonomy*

During endoscopic surgery, an endoscope is inserted into a natural orifice/incision and navigated inside the patient's body, which is a difficult task given the lack of dexterity of the endoscopes available currently. Mechatronics technology can be used to develop highly dexterous or autonomous endoscopes as discussed next.

Dexterous endoscopes   In the tendon-actuated endoscope discussed in [32], the rotational movement is distributed among a number of joints. In this design, it is possible to bend the stem to the desired angle and lock it in that orientation. Compared to the single-joint design, the multi-joint design has the advantages of a wide rotational range and a gradual bend capability although it requires a large space to bend to a desired orientation. Sturges and Laowattana discuss a tendon-actuated bead-chain endoscope [127]. Slatkin et al. have developed a robotic endoscope actuated by inflatable balloons and rubber bellows [123]. Suzumori et al. discuss an electro-hydraulic actuated endoscope whose distal tip can be controlled [130].

Autonomous endoscopes   Some endoscopes are designed to travel through human cavities with greater autonomy. For demanding applications such as colonoscopy, in which a colonoscope is manipulated around a winding colon, autonomous endoscopic devices can be helpful. (Semi-) autonomous crawlers for colonoscopy, angioplasty, inspection of the intestine and colon have been reported in the literature [111, 7]. Devices that crawl in the gastrointestinal (GI) tract and in the colon with shape memory alloy steerable and telescopic tips have been developed [110]. For the GI tract and other tubular organs, other autonomous endoscopes are reported in [62, 123, 143, 99]. In addition to inspection and diagnosis, therapies can also be delivered when miniaturized tools are added to these endoscopes [109].

1.3 Haptics for Robotic Surgery and Therapy

Incorporating haptic sensation to robotic systems for surgery or therapy especially for minimally invasive surgery, which involves limited instrument maneuverability and 2-D camera vision, is a logical next step in the development of these systems. To do so, in addition to instrumentation of surgical tools, appropriate haptics-enabled user interfaces must be developed.

1.3.1 *Haptic user interface technology*

In the following, examples of the currently available haptic devices are described. For a more complete survey of haptic devices, see [55].

1.3.1.1 *PHANToM*

The PHANToM from Sensable Technologies Inc. (www.sensable.com) is one of the most commonly used haptic devices and comes in a number of models with different features. PHANToM 1.5A provides six DOFs input control. Of the six DOFs of the arm, depending on the model, some or all are force-reflective. In Figure 1.2a, a PHANToM 1.5/6DOF with force feedback capability in all of the six DOFs is shown.

1.3.1.2 *Freedom-6S*

The Freedom-6S shown in Figure 1.2b is a 6-DOF device from MPB Technologies Inc. (www.mpb-technologies.ca) that provides force feedback in all of the six degrees of freedom. The position stage is direct driven while the orientation stage is driven remotely by tendons. The Freedom-6S features static and dynamic balancing in all axes (see [54] for further design details).

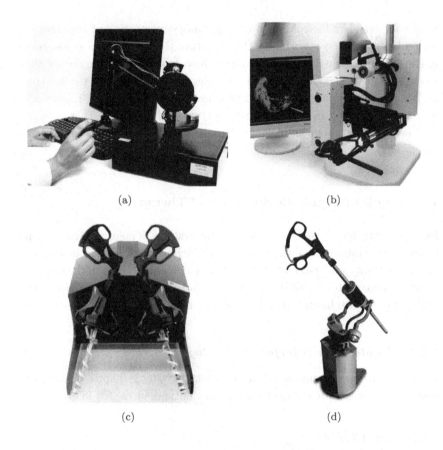

Fig. 1.2 (a) The PHANToM® Premium 1.5/6DOF of Sensable Technologies Inc., (b) the Freedom-6S of MPB Technologies Inc., (c) the Laparoscopic Surgical Workstation of Immersion Corp., and (d) the Xitact IHP of Xitact SA.

1.3.1.3 *Laparoscopic Impulse Engine and Surgical Workstation*

Originally as part of a laparoscopic surgical simulator, the Laparoscopic Impulse Engine was designed by Immersion Corp. (www.immersion.com). The device can track the position of the instrument tip in five DOFs with high resolution and speed while providing force feedback in three DOFs. More recently, Immersion has developed the Laparoscopic Surgical Workstation (Figure 1.2c), which is capable of providing force feedback in five DOFs. An application example is the Virtual Endoscopic Surgery Trainer (VEST) from Select-IT VEST Systems AG (www.select-it.de). The VEST system uses the Laparoscopic Impulse Engine as its force-feedback input interface for simulating laparoscopic surgery interventions.

1.3.1.4   *Xitact IHP*

The Xitact IHP^{TM} from Xitact Medical Simulation (www.xitact.com) is a 4-DOF force feedback manipulator based on a spherical remote-center-of-motion mechanical structure and was originally designed for virtual reality based minimally invasive surgery simulation [42]. It features high output force capability, low friction, zero backlash and a large, singularity-free workspace. A picture of the Xitact IHP is shown in Figure 1.2d.

1.3.2   *Haptic surgical teleoperation*

It has been shown that incorporating force feedback into teleoperated systems can reduce the magnitude of contact forces and therefore the energy consumption, the task completion time and the number of errors. In several studies [122, 147, 15], addition of force feedback is reported to achieve some or all of the following: reduction of the RMS force by 30% to 60%, the peak force by a factor of 2 to 6, the task completion time by 30% and the error rate by 60%.

In [106], a scenario is proposed to incorporate force feedback into the Zeus surgical system by integrating a PHANToM haptic input device into the system. In [85], a dextrous slave combined with a modified PHANToM haptic master which is capable of haptic feedback in four DOFs is presented. A slave system which uses a modified Impulse Engine as the haptic master device is described in [30]. In [107], a telesurgery master-slave system that is capable of reflecting forces in three degrees of freedom (DOFs) is discussed. A master-slave system composed of a 6-DOF parallel slave micromanipulator and a 6-DOF parallel haptic master manipulator is described in [150]. Other examples of haptic surgical teleoperation include [93] and [11]. The haptics technology can also be used for surgical training and simulation purposes. For example, a 7-DOF haptic device that can be applied to surgical training is developed in [56]. A 5-DOF haptic mechanism that is used as part of a training simulator for urological operations is discussed in [146].

1.4   Technological Challenges of the Future

The previous sections presented an overview of the different types of robotic systems for surgery and therapy. Although technological advances mainly in the last two decades have been significant, further improvement in the design and technology of such systems is required for their widespread use. Some of the challenges faced by the field of surgical robotics are as follows.

For providing a surgeon with haptic feedback, the development of specialized, force-reflective user interfaces and the integration of force sensors into surgical robots remain two major challenges. While currently the sterilization requirements are addressed through the use of gas or pre-sterilized drapes to cover the robotic end-effectors, it is necessary to develop actuators and sensors that can go through a relatively inexpensive sterilization process such as autoclaving. Furthermore, to make surgeries less invasive and to facilitate operation in very small spaces such as in pediatric minimally invasive surgery, it is needed to miniaturize the instruments – in the case of pediatric surgery, to less than 3 mm in diameter. It would also be useful to develop intelligent instruments that provide sensory control and guidance, e.g., limit the forces applied to tissue to avoid damage, record hand motions for performance records, or sound alarms when approaching dangerous conditions.

The initial and subsequent costs associated with purchasing and maintaining surgical systems are currently high, limiting the introduction of surgical robots into operating rooms. Such a high cost is mainly due to the highly challenging and lengthy process of obtaining regulatory approval for safety and reliability of a surgical system before it can be commercialized. Optimization and streamlining this process by regulatory agencies and making the surgical systems' software and hardware more modular and standardized can ultimately make the systems cost-effective and affordable.

Chapter 2

Sensorized Surgical Effector (Slave)

2.1 Introduction

With endoscopic surgery, in which an endoscope and endoscopic instruments are inserted into the body cavity through small incisions, the trauma to the body, the post-operative pain and the length of hospital stay are reduced significantly compared to open surgery. However, endoscopic surgery has inherent drawbacks and pitfalls with respect to sensory and motor aspects, as discussed in the following section.

2.1.1 Limitations of endoscopic surgery

The following are some areas in which endoscopic surgery shows limitations:

Observation: The camera platform is unstable and shakes because of the assistant's hand tremor, resulting in visual interruptions and possible motion sickness [8]. Hand-eye coordination is awkward and disorients the surgeon [14] because the relative position and orientation of the endoscope with respect to the instrument does not always match those of the surgeon's eye with respect to his/her hand.

Ergonomics: The surgeon is not in a comfortable position and gets fatigued during surgery [9].

Manipulation: The surgeon's hand tremor is magnified by the long instruments, making it difficult to achieve fine manipulation of objects. The situation is further aggravated by the fact that during endoscopic manipulation the surgeon cannot rest his/her wrist on a surface.

Dexterity: Because the endoscopic instrument pivots about an entry point, it has limited degrees of freedom, hampering fluid rotations of the surgeon's wrist and consequently the dexterity of the motion. This is especially significant when performing complex tasks such as suturing. Experimental motion analysis on suturing and ligating tasks has shown that the mean rotational movements of the brachium and antebrachium and, in particular, the dorsal manus and the instrument are limited in the case of endoscopic manipulation as compared to open surgery, causing the surgeon to extend the translational movements of the brachium and antebrachium as a compensation measure [39].

Tactility/Kinesthesis: The surgeon cannot access the surgical field directly, thereby losing the tactile (cutaneous) perception resulting from direct touch, which is very important in tasks such as tissue palpation or inspection of pulsations. The surgeon has a limited and distorted kinesthetic and force perception of the instrument and its interaction with tissue. The reasons for this are that (1) the cannulae through which instruments are inserted introduce friction, (2) the instrument pivoted at the entry point has a mechanical advantage (ratio of the distances of the two ends of the instrument from the entry point) that varies with the insertion depth, causing the forces at the two ends (resulting from the instrument interaction with the tissue and the hand) to vary and be mismatched as the instrument moves in and out, and (3) the contact forces at the instrument tip can sometimes be negligible compared to the relatively large forces required to move the instrument mass and the unsupported hand and arm [140].

2.1.2 *The need for robot-assisted surgery*

Robots have found extensive use in "assisting" surgical interventions due in part to good stability and geometric accuracy and despite the new challenges they create because of their bulkiness, the required setup time, and the possible collisions of different arms [135, 26, 59, 83]. Using robots and computers to assist in endoscopic surgery is a step toward overcoming some of the difficulties mentioned above. For instance, the problems related to observation are tackled in the following ways:

- In terms of visual steadiness, robotic voice-controlled camera holders can outperform human camera holders without compromising the operation time [71, 105]. Robotic positioners can control the endoscope merely based on the surgeon's facial motions and without verbal, hand or foot commands, paving the way for solo surgery [103].
- With respect to the surgeon's hand-eye coordination, any misori-

entation between the hand movements and the movements on the monitor can be compensated for by a computer.

Moreover, compared to conventional non-robotic endoscopy, robot-assisted endoscopy can be more cost effective [71].

Master-slave robotic surgery   The idea of performing surgery in a master-slave robotic mode, where the movements of a surgical robot (slave) are controlled via a surgeon's console (master), takes robot-assisted surgery into a new era in which robots are given a more significant role. Master-slave robotic operation can solve many of the problems encountered in conventional surgery in the following ways:

Ergonomics: The surgeon becomes less fatigued sitting at a comfortable and ergonomic console while doing endoscopic operations.

Manipulation: Motions of the hand can be scaled down for improved precision. Manipulation can be made even more precise by filtering out natural hand tremors and making both hands equally dominant.

Dexterity: The surgeon's dexterity can be improved by means of articulated wrist-like millirobotic attachments at the end of the instruments [141].

Tactility/Kinesthesis: Any interaction between the instrument and tissue can be reflected to the surgeon's hand by incorporating appropriate sensors and actuators at the patient side and the surgeon side respectively. The contact forces can be scaled up prior to being reflected to the user, in order to make even the smallest contact perceivable to the unsupported hand.

Furthermore, robotic endoscopic surgery can be done with the surgeon operating from a distant location [16].

State of the art   Today's robotic surgical systems (the Zeus and the da Vinci systems [8] – the former is no longer available) provide most of the above-mentioned benefits, but as yet they do not provide feedback of tactile/force (haptic) sensations that are so crucial for the surgeon. The significance of haptic feedback in master-slave operation ("teleoperation" hereafter) is discussed in the following section.

2.1.3   *Significance of haptic perception in master-slave operation*

Transparency of a master-slave system is defined as the extent to which a user feels as if he or she is directly interacting with the environment, while actually performing a task in teleoperation mode. Transparency is a measure of the quality and fidelity of teleoperation which depends on how well the instrument-environment interactions are reflected to the user's hand. In the case of robotic surgery, a fully transparent surgical system mimics human perceptual-motor characteristics to the extent that the surgeon is unable to discriminate between moving the actual surgical instrument and manipulating the console. In other words, for transparency of teleoperation, the master console must provide appropriate force feedback to the user, in order to emulate the environment encountered by the slave-side instrument.

General teleoperation Studies on the effect of force feedback on various object manipulation and target acquisition tasks have revealed that force feedback helps the performance and efficiency of teleoperation by reducing the peak magnitude of contact forces (and trauma to the tissue in the case of surgery), the root-mean-square forces and thus the energy consumption, the task completion time and the number of errors [122, 15]. Study of several object manipulation tasks including peg-in-hole insertions has shown that addition of force feedback achieves reductions in the sum of squared forces by a factor of 7, the task completion time by 30%, and the error rate by 60% [49]. Similarly, analysis of reach-to-grasp movements towards graphic objects in a virtual environment has demonstrated that haptic feedback about object contact is very important for effective interaction between the user and the virtual environment [87]. With the task being the acquisition of a cubic target in a grasp, movement time and peak velocity were improved (i.e., lower and higher respectively) in the presence of haptic feedback. According to Fitt's law [36], the movement time has a direct relationship with the index of difficulty of a motor task and, therefore, a shorter movement time means that haptic feedback has made the task more intuitive. Additionally, there are other studies on the importance of haptic feedback in user interfaces in the context of shortening task completion times and improving perceptional/motor capabilities of the human operator [46, 61].

Robotic surgery Haptic perception, as crucial as it is for teleoperation in general, is even more important in performing surgical tasks where it can affect both the sensory and the motor responses of the surgeon. Haptic feedback can complement sensory modalities such as vision [34] and, therefore, can counterbalance the restricted camera vision in minimally invasive surgery. Haptic feedback can also affect the three main metrics of motor functioning (i.e., precision, speed and force [86]). Haptic feedback, which is important in performing surgical tasks with complex kinematics [34], can enhance the precision when using instruments with restricted or limited maneuverability in minimally invasive surgery. Lack of haptic feedback causes the surgeon to slow down the maneuvers and wait for visual cues as to the strength of the grip, the softness of the tissue, etc., prolonging the operation and hampering the natural and intuitive conduct of the operation. Study of the effect of force feedback on performing blunt dissection [147] has shown that force feedback can reduce the contact forces, the task completion time and the number of errors. Palpation is another procedure frequently used by surgeons to estimate tissue characteristics and locate blood vessels. Without haptic perception and thereby palpation capability, excessive forces may be applied by the surgeon causing complications such as accidental puncturing of blood vessels or tissue damage [129, 51]. Trials on a uni-manual suturing task in a virtual environment has shown that force feedback can reduce the peak force application and the stitch completion time and can improve the "straightness" of the stitch [94]. Moreover, in needle insertion tasks, the ability to detect the puncturing of different tissue layers is improved when users receive haptic feedback [41].

To restore the perception of forces, the surgical instrument needs to be sensorized to measure instrument/tissue interactions. Such an instrument (called the end effector), which is the subject of this chapter, can be used with a surgical robot and a force-reflective console to incorporate force perception in robotic surgery. The applicability of the end effector is discussed further in the following section.

2.1.4 *Perceptual-motor skills study*

The use of the sensorized end effector developed in this chapter is not limited to providing haptic feedback during robotic surgery. It can also be used for research purposes, for example, to study the sensory and motor skills of residents and surgeons.

In endoscopic manipulation, the reduced dexterity, the loss of direct contact with organs and tactile sensation, and the significant degradation in the force sensation result in new perceptual-motor relationships which are unfamiliar and must be learned [139]. The required perceptual-motor skills take longer than normal to master and pose a learning challenge to surgeons interested in the development of these skills. An endoscopic end effector, which measures the force/torque data resulting from interactions with tissue, can be exploited to objectively assess the skill level and the learning curve of a user. Novice and experienced surgeons leave quite different force/torque and temporal statistical signatures (including force/torque magnitudes and time intervals for various instrument/tissue interactions) while manipulating and dissecting tissue [113]. The sensorized end effector discussed in this chapter can be used with a surgical robotic system (even without a force-reflection capability) as a training tool to help surgical residents learn how to best exert forces and torques on tissue in various surgical maneuvers and scenarios and correct any problems that may arise.

2.2   Methods, Materials and Results

To provide the surgeon with force perception during robotic endoscopic surgery, the following two devices are needed at the patient and surgeon sides:

- An endoscopic surgical instrument that acts as the last arm (end effector) of the slave surgical robot and is properly sensorized to measure instrument/tissue interactions in the form of forces or moments.
- A force-reflective human-machine interface that mediates between the surgeon and the robot, transferring hand movement commands to the robot and instrument/tissue interaction measurements to the surgeon's hand.

Our research concerns restoring force (and moment) feedback to the surgeon. Tactile feedback, which involves stimulation of cutaneous receptors to perceive mechanical, thermal and other cutaneous stimuli at the skin surface, is a much more difficult task. While some research is underway to develop tactile sensors for minimally invasive surgery [70], the lack of a human-machine interface that effectively displays cutaneous stimuli to the hand is a significant impediment. In this chapter, we discuss a robotic endoscopic end effector that measures any force/moment interaction it has through contact with its environment.

2.2.1 *Force reflection methods*

In principle, force feedback in a master-slave system is possible even without force sensing at the slave side. In fact, a real-time control algorithm minimizing the position/orientation difference between the master and the slave manipulators can provide some force sensation to the user manipulating the master. However, as suggested in [121], this position error-based force reflection scheme accounts for an inferior teleoperation performance (transparency) as compared to force reflection using a force sensor at the slave side. Additionally, the perception of forces is sluggish and delayed.

To explore the above further, we set up an experiment in which two PHANToM haptic devices act as the master and the slave, and are controlled using the position-error based scheme. The setup was used to qualitatively examine whether the palpation of soft objects can be done effectively using this method of force reflection. Our experiments showed that a low-stiffness object is compliant with the slave robot position changes, causing the position error to be always small. Since the force reflected to the user is proportional to the position error, in order to have a perceivable force feedback, the corresponding gain should be high. A high gain, however, causes some force to be reflected to the hand even with the slave robot moving in free space due to any control inaccuracies. Lowering the gain to solve this problem introduces another problem: The user may damage the tissue by incurring excessive deformations because insufficient forces are being transmitted to the user's hand. Therefore, with a tradeoff on the controller gain, the dynamic range of perceivable forces is limited.

The surgeon's console of the da Vinci surgical system has force feedback capability in some degrees of freedom. This force feedback, however, is unrealistic and of low quality and therefore has been disabled. The main reason is that no force sensing capability is present at the end effector of the robot; instead the contact forces are estimated from outside the patient. The unwanted consequences of the estimation of contacts from outside the patient are picking up disturbance forces caused by the port through which the instrument is inserted, and biased and noisy force feedback.

Apart from the above, other techniques for master-slave force reflection share a common need for slave-side force measurement [121, 80]. With such techniques and with an end effector properly sensorized to measure all interactions it has with the tissue from inside the patient, the adverse effects of sensorless force feedback are excluded from the haptic teleoperation loop.

2.2.2 *Design requirements*

Developing a robotic end effector that is sensorized and actuated in accordance with the requirements of endoscopic surgery is not easy. Due to the constraint on incision size in endoscopic surgery, the diameter of the robotic end effector including all required sensors as well as the tip actuator should be less than 10 mm. Here is a list of issues to be considered in designing a robotic endoscopic end effector:

- The currently available multi-axis sensors that measure forces and torques in all six degrees of freedom (three translational and three rotational) are at least about twice as wide and, therefore, have to stay outside the patient. A miniature force sensor that is 12.5 mm in diameter and is intended for measuring small contact forces at the tip of a microsurgical instrument is the subject of a recent research work [10]; however, it is only capable of measuring forces in three dimensions. Being located outside the patient causes the sensors to pick up unwanted abdominal wall friction and stiffness at the trocar site[1], causing distortions in the sensation of forces.
- Due to the limited amount of space, the pivotal motions of the tip jaws (e.g. grasper jaws) need to be actuated by a linear motion, preferably placed outside the patient. This also poses another challenge related to the previous requirement: if a force sensor is used, it must be hollow to accommodate the rod whose linear motions actuate the tip.
- The sensor measuring the interactions between the tip and the tissue should not be mounted directly on the tip jaws because, for sterilizability reasons, it is desirable to use tips that can be detached and disposed of after use.

We tackle the first problem by non-invasive measurements of interactions using strain gauges that are integrated into the endoscopic end effector. For the second and third requirements, a mechanism consisting of a linear motor and a load cell is used to non-invasively actuate a detachable tip and measure its interactions with tissue.

---

[1]A trocar (usually used with a cannula) is a hollow tube introduced through a tiny incision in the abdominal or chest wall. In endoscopic surgery, a surgeon gains entry to the body cavity through the trocar and the cannula.

2.2.3 Twist and tip motions

Twist motion and free wrist Regardless of the kinematic properties of a surgical robot, a mechanism for the roll motion (twist about the main axis) of the end effector is needed. In Figure 2.1a, a geared motor/encoder combination[2] responsible for twisting the instrument is placed at the base of the assembly. A wrist (made by links L_1, L_2 and L_3 in Figure 2.1a) is attached to the roll motor and is built such that if the motor faces resistance while trying to rotate the instrument (and the tissue), the wrist will not twist into itself. This is simply because the axes of the motor and the joint connecting links L_1 and L_2 do not ever align in the workspace ($-90° <$ yaw angle $< 90°$). The reason for having the wrist is given in Section 2.3.

Tip actuation The tools used in endoscopic surgery to grasp or cut tissue have their jaws pivotally moved relative to one another by a linear motion actuator. For the end effector developed here, the elements of the tip actuation assembly (open/close motion) as well as two detachable scissors and grasper tips are shown in Figure 2.1b. There are three concentric tubes – outer, middle and inner. The inner tube is displaced with respect to the middle one by a linear motor (Zaber Technologies Inc.), in order to control the tip jaws. The reason for having an additional outer tube is discussed in Section 2.2.4. Figures 2.1c and 2.1d show an exploded view of the overall end effector and a section view of the tip actuation assembly.

Tip model To control the jaw's angular position, it is necessary to find its relationship with the linear displacement that actuates it. The sketch of an atraumatic forceps tip (Fundus grasper 3211, Microline Inc.) in two different positions is shown in Figure 2.2. Here, $\alpha = \theta + \alpha_0$ and the jaw angle θ can be found from the linear displacement x as

$$\sin(\theta + \alpha_0) = \frac{L}{D - x} \tag{2.1}$$

Tip model identification The parameters α_0, L and D of equation (2.1) for the specified tool tip have to be found empirically. An experiment was set up in which the linear motor moved the tip to 30 positions (corresponding to the angle between the two jaws of the tip ranging from 0 to 63°) and the linear position x as well as the angle 2θ were registered. Then, a

---

[2]The graphite-brush DC motor model RE25-118752, the 500 CPT quadrature encoder with line driver HEDL 5540 model 110512, and the 84:1 reduction planetary gearhead model 144039, all from Maxon Precision Motors, Inc.

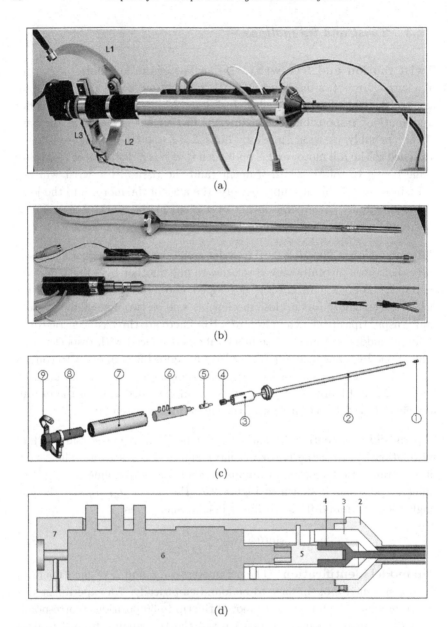

Fig. 2.1   (a) The overall end effector including the wrist, twist motor and tip actuation assembly, (b) details of the tip actuation assembly: the three tubes and two different detachable tips, (c) an exploded view of (a), and (d) a section view of (b). In (c) and (d): (1) tip, (2) outer tube, (3) middle tube, (4) inner tube, (5) load cell, (6) linear motor, (7) outer housing, (8) twist motor, and (9) free wrist.

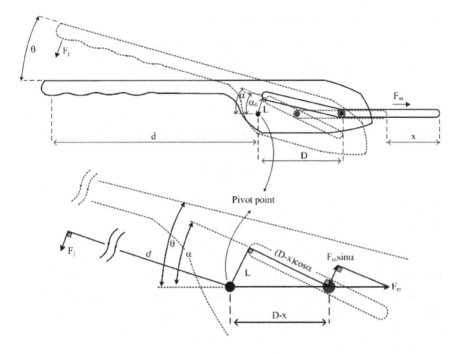

Fig. 2.2   Surgical grasper mechanism and a close-up.

Table 2.1   Grasper tip parameter estimates.

	Mean	Standard deviation / Mean
α_0	25.15°	2.1 %
L	2.34 mm	3.9 %
D	5.91 mm	1.7 %

nonlinear minimization (Gauss-Newton method) was used to find the values for α_0, L and D that best satisfied equation (2.1). The mean values for the resulting parameter estimates obtained using four trials are listed in Table 2.1. A consistency measure has been defined as the ratio of the standard deviation of the estimates to their mean value. Small consistency measures for the estimated parameters promise a good match with the actual values. The value of d was separately determined to be 22 mm.

2.2.4   Interaction measurement

Having obtained the position model of the tip (equation (2.1)), we need to determine the force model. From Figure 2.2, the balance of moments about the pivot point leads to

$$F_j d = (F_m \sin \alpha)((D - x) \cos \alpha).$$

Using equation (2.1) and $\alpha = \theta + \alpha_0$, the following force propagation model is obtained:

$$F_j = F_m \frac{L \cos(\theta + \alpha_0)}{d} \tag{2.2}$$

Equation (2.2) demonstrates that it is possible to determine the tip/tissue interaction F_j, which is due to the open/close motions of the jaws, based on the linear tension/compression F_m measurable by a single-axis load cell. Using the parameter estimates of Table 2.1, the nonlinear relationship between F_m/F_j and the jaw angle θ is depicted in Figure 2.3. A miniature load cell[3] was attached between the linear motor shaft and the inner tube (Figure 2.4a) so that equation (2.2) can be used to extract the interaction forces of the jaws with the environment based on the linear tension/compression measured by the load cell.

Possible maneuvers of the instrument involve lateral and axial force interactions at the distal end, occurring when pushing or pulling on tissue, and torsional moment interactions that can happen, for example, during suturing. Assuming that the instrument axis is defined by z, the instrument endpoint forces (f_x f_y f_z) and the twist moment τ_z can be determined from the measurements of all moments (τ_x τ_y τ_z) and the axial force f_z, provided that interactions only occur at the end point of the instrument. Several strain gauges are used to non-invasively measure all of these interactions with the tissue:

- Strain gauges are placed on opposite sides of the surface of the outer tube such that any lateral force at the endpoint causes tension in one strain gauge and compression in the other (Figure 2.4b). These full-bridged gauges register the two bending moments τ_x and τ_y.
- Compressional/tensional axial force f_z is registered by the full-bridged strain gauges placed on a link of the 2-dof wrist (Fig-

---

[3]Load cell XFTC-101-M5F from FGP Sensors and Instrumentation, which is 10 mm in diameter and has a measurement range of 20 N in tension and compression. The transducer has been optimized at low ranges and has a combined hysteresis and nonlinearity of less than $\pm 0.5\%$ full-scale.

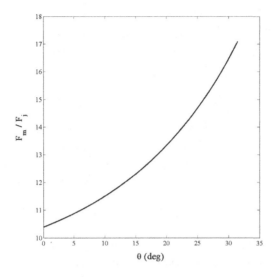

Fig. 2.3 The ratio of axial and tip forces vs. the jaw angle.

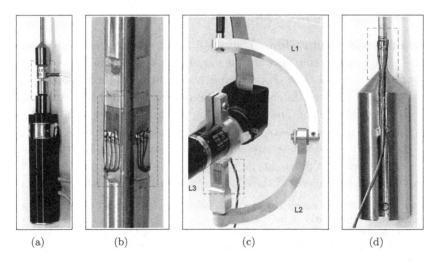

Fig. 2.4 (a) load cell to find tip forces, (b) gauges to measure bending moments, (c) gauges to measure the axial forces, and (d) gauge to measure the torsional moment.

Table 2.2   Voltage vs. axial force relationship parameter estimates.

		Mean	$\frac{\text{Standard deviation}}{\text{Mean}}$
Compression	α	2.58×10^{-1}	5.5%
	β	-7.09×10^{-1}	8.1%
Tension	α	3.48×10^{-1}	4.5%
	β	-1.48×10^{-1}	31.8%

ure 2.4c). This wrist is responsible for allowing the spherical motions of the end effector centered at the entry point through the skin (see Section 2.3).

- The twist moment τ_z is measured by the torque gauge on the middle tube (Figure 2.4d) as the tip's outer body threads onto it.

Note that each of the above strain gauges, supplied by Intertechnology Inc.[4], is in a transverse arrangement with respect to others such that the cross-talk between them is reduced as much as possible.

The reason for having three tubes in the end effector assembly becomes clear here. This arrangement isolates the differential force exerted for actuating the tip from measurements in the other directions. More specifically, the middle tube, which floats between the inner and outer tubes, prevents the differential inner/middle tube force from affecting the strain gauges mounted on the outer tube for measuring lateral forces.

Strain gauge calibration   The strain gauges are calibrated by finding the (linear) relationship between the output voltages and the forces/torques applied at the tool tip[5]. For example, to calibrate the axial force gauge shown in Figure 2.4c, different masses were attached to the assembly held in the vertical position and the resulting voltage readings were recorded. In this particular case, there is a no-load voltage present due to the weight of the motor. The least-squares method was used to find a line that best describes these data points in the voltage versus axial force plane. Table 2.2 shows the mean values and the consistency measures (the ratio of standard

---

[4]For the bending moments and the axial forces, the EA-06-062-TV-350 gauge with a gauge factor (the ratio of fractional change in electrical resistance to the fractional change in length) of $2.045 \pm 0.5\%$ and a cross-sensitivity of $(1.4 \pm 0.2)\%$ was used. For the twist moment, the EA-06-125PC-350 gauge with a nominal gauge factor of 2.090 was used.

[5]One SGA/D Strain Gage Amplifier from Magna Projects and Instruments Ltd. was used for each channel. It provides an adjustable transducer sensitivity between 0.06 to 30.3 mV/V and user-selectable analogue output options $\pm$10V, $\pm$5V, 0-10V, 0-5V, 0-20mA, and 4-20mA and several filtering options.

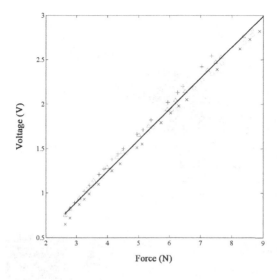

Fig. 2.5 The experimental $V - f_z$ data points for the four experiments (plus, cross, triangle, circle) and the least-squares linear fit (solid line) during tension.

deviation to mean) of the parameter estimates α and β in $V = \alpha f_z + \beta$ where V is the voltage readout and f_z is the axial compression or tension force. Figure 2.5 shows the data points for the four experiments where the assembly has been under tension (the shifted origin is due the weight of the motor) and the linear fit is as shown in Table 2.2. The calibration of the other strain gauges is done in a similar manner.

2.3 Discussion

The endoscopic end effector can be used with or without the free wrist (made by links L_1, L_2 and L_3 in Figure 2.1a) depending on the kinematic properties of the surgical robot. With the wrist, the end effector can be used with any robot that provides positioning in 3-D space and with a fulcrum placed at the trocar to form a constrained isocenter. The fulcrum supports the end effector so that its movements do not damage the tissue near the trocar. Without the wrist, the end effector should be used with a robot that provides spherical movement at a Remote Center of Motion (RCM) located at the entry point. As the motion sequence for the da Vinci robot shows

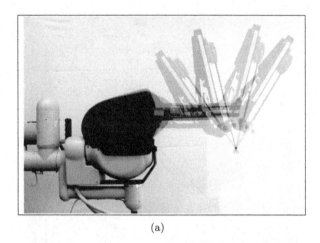

(a)

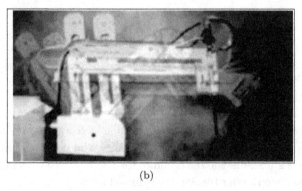

(b)

Fig. 2.6   The remote center of motion (RCM) created by (a) the da Vinci and (b) the Neurobot © 2002 IEEE.

(Figure 2.6a), the RCM-based manipulator can provide two rotations (yaw and pitch) and one translation (in/out) centered at a fixed point along the instrument (coincident with the entry point), such that the instrument tip can be positioned anywhere inside a cone. Most of the robots that provide an RCM do so by a parallelogram mechanism that simulates a spherical joint at the entry point, e.g., as shown in Figure 2.6b for the Neurobot [27]. A summary of surgical robotic systems and their characteristics including the number of degrees of freedom and whether they provide an RCM is given in [135]. Recent advances in active constraints technology for creating an RCM are discussed in [125].

When using the end effector in a master-slave system, an issue to consider is how to use the tip's position and force models. In a hand-held endoscopic instrument, there is a difference between the tip angular position (or force interaction) and the handle angular position (or force interaction). For example, in a Carl Storz Babcock grasper tool, there is a gain of 1.2 between the angular positions of the tip and the handpiece while the transfer function between the interactions (force/moment) is more involved [115]. In a robotic master-slave setting, where the surgical end-effector's tip is controlled by a handle at the surgeon's console, it is important to preserve the same tip/handle relationships (in terms of position and force) to minimize the perceptual and motor mappings that an endoscopic surgeon would have to learn to perform robotic endoscopic surgery.

2.4 Concluding Remarks

The incorporation of haptic feedback is a logical next stage for robotic surgical systems. It makes robotic surgery and therapy more efficient, accurate and reliable, and the surgeon's task more intuitive. The endoscopic robotic end effector presented in this chapter is capable of measuring tool/tissue interaction in all five degrees of freedom present in endoscopic operations (pitch, yaw, roll, insertion and gripping). Indeed, the three-stage instrument assembly and its strain gauge sensors provide a non-invasive, efficient solution to the problems posed by the incision size constraint in minimally invasive surgery. The end effector features the non-invasive actuation of a detachable tip and the measurement of tip interaction forces (grasping, cutting, etc.) without using sensors on the jaws.

The end effector is capable of using disposable, detachable tips of all functionalities (www.microlineinc.com). Thin wires running from the strain gauges measuring lateral forces (Figure 2.4b) back to the base of the end effector can be placed in the tiny groves made on the shaft surface and then covered by a sterilized coat, or they can run inside the instrument in the space between the outer and the middle tubes. All other wires are far from the tip of the instrument. Nevertheless, the sterilizability of the end-effector needs to be considered more fully before it is used in clinical trials.

The sensorized end effector and the free wrist discussed in this chapter are used at the slave side of a robotic master-slave test-bed for studying haptics-based interaction in a minimally invasive environment (Figure 2.7). The PHANToM haptic device used on the slave side acts merely as a robotic

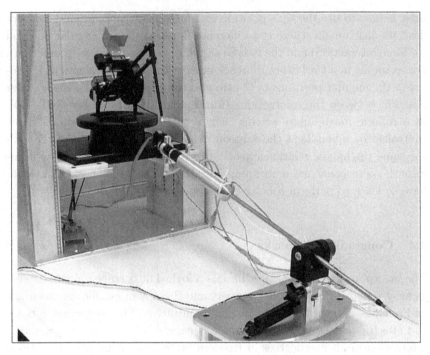

Fig. 2.7   The slave subsystem of a master-slave test-bed for a minimally invasive surgery environment.

manipulator as no force reflection is involved at the slave side. The user is able to manipulate the master, described in the next chapter, causing the slave to execute a desired motion of the endoscopic instrument. The user receives haptic feedback via the master interface. The developed master-slave system is a useful test-bed to investigate the performance and effectiveness of different master-slave control schemes. The system can be tested under different circumstances in which it is expected to operate, for example, with varying tissue properties and different ranges of applied forces. The Virtual Reality Peripheral Network (VRPN) [138] has been used to establish network-based communication between the master and slave subsystems so that the slave can be telemanipulated by the user sitting at the master console at a distant location. Therefore, the system is also useful in exploring the effects of communication latency on the stability and performance of the haptics-based master-slave system and finding ways to compensate for time delay in a real-time, human-in-the-loop telemanipulation. For more information about the slave system discussed in this chapter, see Appendix A.

Chapter 3

Haptic User Interface (Master)

3.1 Introduction

In force-reflective master-slave teleoperation, the surgeon operates from and receives force feedback via a master interface while a slave robot mimics the surgeon's hand maneuvers on the patient's body. Similarly, in a virtual-reality environment, the user manipulates virtual and usually deformable objects and receives force feedback through an interface similar to the master interface in master-slave robotic surgery. It was discussed in Chapter 2 how haptic feedback at the surgeon's console of a robot-assisted surgical system can improve the performance and efficiency of operation. Alternatively, the same human-machine interface can be used in computer-assisted surgical simulation and training to create the perception of interaction with the virtual environment for the user. The following section discusses how this can make surgical training more efficient and realistic.

3.1.1 *Computer-assisted endoscopic surgery training*

In endoscopic surgery, the limitations on the degrees of freedom and the surgeon's dexterity, the loss of the tactile sensation, and the significant degradation in the force sensation result in new perceptual-motor relationships which are unfamiliar and require training [139]. In conventional training, the trainee first watches a skilled professional do an operation and then cooperates with the professional in doing the task. In the case of training for endoscopic surgery, however, the required perceptual-motor skills take longer than normal to master and pose a challenge to surgeons. A possible solution to this learning problem is computer-assisted surgical simulation with unique advantages such as the possibility of repeated practice. The

Minimally Invasive Surgery Trainer (MIST^{TM}) from Mentice Corporation (www.mentice.com) is an example of computer-assisted simulators, which has also been validated through clinical trials [131]. Some trainers have been equipped with haptic feedback, e.g., the Virtual Endoscopic Surgery Trainer from Select-IT VEST Systems AG (www.select-it.de). The efficiency of computer-assisted interactive training environments can be improved by haptic feedback as discussed in the following section.

3.1.1.1   *Haptic perception in computer-assisted surgical training*

Analysis of reach-to-grasp movements towards graphic objects in a virtual environment has demonstrated that haptic feedback about object contact can decrease movement time and increase peak velocity [87]. This is important because, according to Fitt's law [36], movement time has a direct relationship with the index of difficulty of a motor task. There are other studies on the benefits of haptic feedback in virtual-reality simulations in terms of shortening task completion times and improving perceptual/motor capabilities of the human operator [46, 61]. Similarly, virtual-reality based surgical training can be improved by haptic feedback [22]. In particular, haptic feedback can be of special importance in learning to perform surgical tasks with complex kinematics. Trials on a uni-manual suturing task in a virtual environment have shown that force feedback can reduce the peak force application and the stitch completion time and can improve the straightness of the stitch [94].

In endoscopic surgery, the prolonged learning period for perceptual-motor skills is partly due to the fact that the perspective is not updated with the surgeon's head movements, thereby disrupting the hand-eye coordination. A study done in a virtual environment using Fitt's tapping task, in which subjects tap back and forth between two objects, has shown that force feedback can improve performance regardless of the perspective [6]. Similarly, in endoscopic surgery training, force feedback may assist the surgeon's adaptation to an incorrect viewpoint (through re-calibration of the eye-to-hand mapping) and accelerate the learning process.

Another computer-assisted, haptics-based surgical training approach, called "haptic guidance", involves physically guiding a trainee through the desired motion by haptic feedback from the user interface, thus helping the trainee to gain an objective kinesthetic understanding of the task required [34].

As discussed in Chapter 2, the following two devices are needed at the surgeon and patient sides for haptics-based endoscopic operation: (1) A force-reflective surgeon-robot interface that transmits hand movements to the slave surgical robot and instrument/tissue interactions to the surgeon's hand. (2) An endoscopic instrument that acts as the last arm (end-effector) of the slave robot and is properly sensorized to measure instrument/tissue interactions in the form of forces or torques. While (2) was the topic of Chapter 2, this chapter is organized as follows to discuss (1). A force-reflective user interface appropriate for an endoscopic surgery environment is discussed in Section 3.2. Mathematical methods for performance analysis and optimization of the force-reflective interface based on the Jacobian matrix of the interface and its singular values are proposed in Section 3.3. Section 3.4 has the concluding remarks.

3.2 Haptic User Interface Architecture

The desirable features of a haptic device for accurate force reflection are very low backdrive friction particularly for low-impedance environments, low inertia, low backlash in the transmission as it introduces discontinuity in the transmitted forces, the capability for large force reflections, and a large force feedback bandwidth. To design a haptic device, the anatomical and physiological features of the human body, particularly the hand and fingers, must also be taken into account. We consider the following important factors pertaining to the hardware and software design of a force-reflective user interface: (1) A virtual surface with a stiffness of at least 20 N/cm or a resisting force of at least 11 N is perceived as solid and immovable by users [88]. (2) Human fingers can sense absolute and relative force variations of 0.5 N and ±7%, respectively [122]. The first factor determines the maximum force that the device may be required to reflect (e.g., to create the perception of hitting a bone in the case of surgical applications). The second feature determines the minimum precision that the force measurements and the force reflection should have.

The possible DOFs for an endoscopic instrument excluding the tip's motions are only four: up and down rotation (pitch), side to side rotation (yaw), axial rotation (roll), and axial translation (insertion). The developed haptic interface is configured to have the same DOFs as conventional endoscopic surgery to provide a natural feel to the surgeon. As a result, the geometric relationships and motor skills for which an endoscopic surgeon is trained are preserved. This is important because robotic endoscopic surgery is shown to require more skills on the part of surgeons and involve a slow learning curve [58]. Therefore, it is helpful to have a user interface that favors exploiting the surgeon's past cognitive and motor skills while bringing about the unique advantages of robot-assisted surgery (e.g. scaling up instrument/tissue interactions prior to reflection to the user's hand, scaling down and/or filtering hand motions). Also as a result of maintaining the same DOFs, the developed user interface is the appropriate platform for exploring the effect of haptic feedback on the particular type of hand-eye coordination problems present during endoscopic surgery. While haptic feedback has been shown to reduce the effect of hand-eye mismatch due to a wrong perspective (see Section 3.1.1.1), it still remains to be seen if it can counterbalance the hand-eye mapping distortions due to the reverse motions of endoscopic instruments pivoted at the incision point.

A possible arrangement for the haptic interface is shown in Figure 3.1. This haptic feedback device is capable of providing the user with force sensation, sensation regarding surface roughness, and kinesthetic sensation of the elasticity of an object. The developed user interface is haptics-enabled in all the regular four DOFs in addition to the finger loops motions. The low cost of this haptic user interface, which can be interfaced to another robot or a computer simulation depending on the application, makes it a reasonable choice for training applications where the use of an expensive, full-blown surgical system may not be economically justifiable. Below, we explain reflecting forces/torques in each of the DOFs available during endoscopic manipulation.

3.2.1   *Force reflection in pitch, yaw and insertion*

The PHANToM 1.5A , which provides force feedback and position measurement at its end point in three translational DOFs, is integrated into the user interface (the PHANToM's stylus has been removed as it has only passive motions). A rigid shaft resembling an endoscopic instrument is passed through a fulcrum and attached to the PHANToM's endpoint, causing the motions of the handles grasped by the surgeon to be similar to those in endoscopic manipulation. The 3-D Cartesian workspace of the PHANToM spans the pitch, yaw and insertion motions of the instrument, thus providing force feedback and position measurement in these three DOFs for the endoscopic instrument.

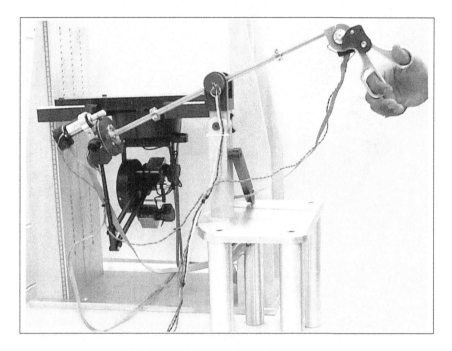

Fig. 3.1   Haptic user interface for endoscopic interventions.

3.2.2   *Force reflection in roll and gripping*

There is a need to incorporate additional mechanisms for force reflection in
the roll and gripping directions. Single-DOF force feedback mechanisms are
used to establish force reflection in each of these directions[1] (Figure 3.2).
The modularity of the interface allows the components to be used in different applications. For example, in a needle insertion scenario, in which the
user pushes the needle while rotating it, one can use the finger loops and the
roll mechanism to control the insertion depth and the twist of the needle,
respectively. The design specifications discussed previously are considered
in the choice of transmission and motor for the single-DOF haptic devices.

Choice of transmission

Due to the requirement of large force reflections, use of a direct-drive motor
is not an option. On the other hand, as studied earlier with regard to

---

[1]These two mechanisms have been intentionally placed on opposite sides of the fulcrum
in order to have as much static balancing as possible.

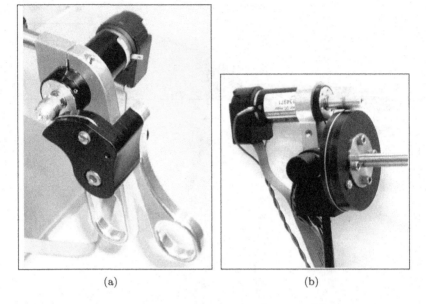

(a)   (b)

Fig. 3.2   Single-DOF force reflection in (a) the finger loops, and (b) the roll mechanism.

the PHANToM device, gear reductions involve significant backlash while a cogless cable-capstan transmission can provide a low-friction, zero-backlash drive for speed reduction and torque amplification [88]. Thus, in each of the single-DOF haptic devices in Figure 3.2, a pre-tensioned cable[2] pinned at two points on the (sector) disk and wrapped several times around the motor pulley implements a cable-capstan transmission. In Figure 3.2a, the motor is secured to the fixed handle and, through a cable transmission of 3.5 : 1, rotates the other handle fixed to the sector disk. This can lead to application of forces against the squeezing thumb of the user depending on the torque supplied by the motor. Similarly, in Figure 3.2b, the motor is fixed with respect to the PHANTOM's last link and, through a cable transmission of 7 : 1, twists the disk and the instrument attached to it thus applying torques in the twist direction on the user's hand.

For each motor, a 500 CPT quadrature encoder (HEDL 5540 with line driver from Maxon Precision Motors, Inc.) is used. Assuming that the cable-capstan transmissions introduce no backlash, the position tracking

---

[2]Uncoated 7 × 19 construction 0.018 diameter stainless steel aircraft cable.

Table 3.1 Specifications of the motor in the single-DOF haptic devices.

	Motor data	Unit
Assigned power rating	20	W
No load speed	9550	rpm
Stall torque	243	mNm
Max continuous torque	26.1	mNm
Rotor inertia	10.3	gcm^2

resolution in the roll and gripping directions are calculated as

$$\text{Resolution}_{\text{Roll}} = \frac{1}{2}\frac{360°/(4 \times 500)}{7/1} = 0.013°$$

$$\text{Resolution}_{\text{Gripping}} = \frac{1}{2}\frac{360°/(4 \times 500)}{3.5/1} = 0.025°$$

Choice of motor

For haptic applications, brushed DC motors are preferred over brushless motors, which suffer from the reluctance cogging and torque ripple phenomena. An appropriate brushed DC motor with low inertia and friction (model RE25-118752, Maxon Precision Motors, Inc.) is selected. Table 3.1 summarizes the specifications of the motor used in the single-DOF haptic devices.

To be able to produce large forces, the stall torque for the motor is the primary specification. Given the distance d_{endpoint} between the effector point and the motor shaft, the transmission ratio n given above, and the desired maximum exertable force F_{max} specified previously, the minimum required peak torque for the motor was found from

$$\tau_{\text{stall}} = \frac{F_{\text{max}} \times d_{\text{endpoint}}}{n}. \tag{3.1}$$

3.3 Analysis of the Haptic Interface

In order to analyze or optimize the haptic interface in terms of sensitivity to positioning errors, workspace, conditioning, and force reflection capability, the Jacobian matrix of the haptic interface is derived first. As discussed in Appendix C, the PHANToM measures the position of its endpoint with respect to the home position defined by a fixed base frame $\{B\}$ in Figure 3.3.

The PHANToM's forward kinematics in the base frame are written as:

$$x = s_1(\ell_1 c_2 + \ell_2 s_3)$$
$$y = \ell_2 - \ell_2 c_3 + \ell_1 s_2 \qquad (3.2)$$
$$z = -\ell_1 + c_1(\ell_1 c_2 + \ell_2 s_3)$$

where $s_i = \sin(\theta_i)$ and $c_i = \cos(\theta_i)$, $i = 1, 2, 3$, $X = (x, y, z)$ is the Cartesian position of the endpoint E with respect to the base frame, and $\Theta = (\theta_1, \theta_2, \theta_3)$ is the PHANToM's motor position vector. In practice, due to an attachment which connects the PHANToM's endpoint to the endoscopic instrument endpoint, the length of the second arm of the PHANToM is increased to $\hat{\ell}_2 = \ell_2 + a$. Therefore, the position of the new endpoint $\tilde{E}$ with respect to the new base frame $\{\tilde{B}\}$ (denoted $^{\tilde{B}}X_{\tilde{E}}$) is found by replacing ℓ_2 by $\hat{\ell}_2$ in equations (3.2). To find the position of the handle of the endoscopic instrument H, we express all positions with respect to a fixed frame $\{F\}$ at the fulcrum. In the following, d and β define the relative position and angle of the PHANToM's base with respect to the fulcrum's base ($\beta = 0$ in the configuration shown in Figure 3.3), and L is the length of the endoscopic instrument.

$$^F_{\tilde{B}}T = \begin{pmatrix} \sin\beta & 0 & -\cos\beta & d \\ 0 & -1 & 0 & 0 \\ -\cos\beta & 0 & -\sin\beta & 0 \\ 0 & 0 & 0 & 1 \end{pmatrix}$$

$$^F X_{\tilde{E}} = {}^F_{\tilde{B}}T\, {}^{\tilde{B}}X_{\tilde{E}}$$

$$^F X_{\tilde{H}} = {}^F X_{\tilde{E}}\left(1 - \frac{L}{\|{}^F X_{\tilde{E}}\|_2}\right) \qquad (3.3)$$

For a robot, the Jacobian matrix J, which relates the endpoint Cartesian positions to the joint angles as $\dot{X} = J\dot{\Theta}$, can be determined by differentiating the forward kinematics with respect to time. Therefore, using equations (3.2), the Jacobian of the PHANToM in the base frame is

$$J_{\mathrm{PH}}(\Theta) = \begin{pmatrix} c_1(\ell_1 c_2 + \ell_2 s_3) & -\ell_1 s_1 s_2 & \ell_2 s_1 c_3 \\ 0 & \ell_1 c_2 & \ell_2 s_3 \\ -s_1(\ell_1 c_2 + \ell_2 s_3) & -\ell_1 c_1 s_2 & \ell_2 c_1 c_3 \end{pmatrix} \qquad (3.4)$$

Also, using (3.3), the haptic interface Jacobian $J(\Theta, d, \beta, L)$ in frame $\{F\}$ is found, but not shown here. For analysis purposes, we will need the following theorem as well:

Theorem 3.1. *For any vectors p and q related through a Jacobian relationship $q = \hat{J}p$, if $\|p\| = 1$ where $\|.\|$ denotes the 2-norm of a vector, then*

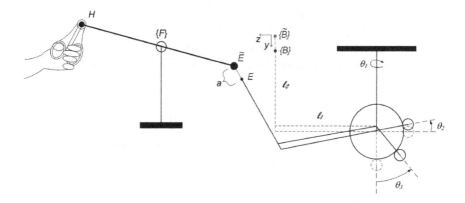

Fig. 3.3   The sketch of the haptic interface.

$\|q_{\min}\| = \sigma_{\min}$ *and* $\|q_{\max}\| = \sigma_{\max}$ *where* $\sigma_{\min}$ *and* $\sigma_{\max}$ *are respectively the smallest and largest singular values of the matrix* $\hat{J}$ *[40].*

3.3.1   *Sensitivity*

The first characteristic of the haptic interface that is analyzed here is the fidelity of the force feedback provided by the PHANToM. In the PHANToM, the motor torque τ required to produce a desired force F at the endpoint is calculated as $F = (J_{\mathrm{PH}}^{\mathrm{T}}(\Theta))^{-1}\tau \doteq J_F(\Theta)\tau$. The issue is that the PHANToM's encoders measure positions relative to the position upon restart (called the zero position). Therefore, any offset between the zero position and the home position assumed in the forward kinematics and the Jacobian causes erroneous θ_i measurements and consequently a deviation between the intended force and the actual force reflected to the user.

To explore this further, assume that there is some small offset error δ in all encoder measurements, i.e. $\tilde{\theta}_i = \theta_i + \delta$, where $\tilde{\theta}_i$ and θ_i, $i = 1, 2, 3$, are the measured and actual positions, respectively. The intended and actual force feedback at the endpoint are related to the motor torque vector τ by $\tilde{F} = J_F(\theta_i + \delta)\tau$ and $F = J_F(\theta_i)\tau$, respectively. We define the normalized force feedback error as

$$\eta = \frac{\|\tilde{F} - F\|_2}{\|F\|_2} \tag{3.5}$$

where $\|.\|$ is the vector 2-norm, and try to determine how the initial positioning error δ affects the force feedback error η. Since δ (rad) is small, a

Taylor series expansion around θ_i yields $J_F(\theta_i + \delta) \approx J_F(\theta_i) + \delta J^1(\theta_i)$. As a result, $\eta = |\delta| \cdot \|J^1 \tau\|_2 / \|J_F \tau\|_2$. Assuming without loss of generality that $\|\tau\|_2 = 1$, Theorem 3.1 can be used to conclude that:

(1) To have a normalized force feedback error $\eta \le \eta_1$, the initial angle error δ_0 must satisfy

$$|\delta_0| \le \eta_1 \min_{\text{workspace}} \frac{\sigma_{\max}(J_F)}{\sigma_{\min}(J^1)}.$$

(2) For a given initial angle offset δ_0, the normalized force feedback error is bounded at each point within the workspace as

$$\eta \le |\delta_0| \frac{\sigma_{\max}(J^1)}{\sigma_{\min}(J_F)}. \tag{3.6}$$

For the PHANToM, equation (3.6) is used to find the upper bound on the normalized force feedback error η per $1°$ initial angle error. Since the value of η varies across the three dimensional workspace of the device, only the iso-value contours of η on three orthogonal planes (corresponding to $x = 0$, $y = 0$ and $z = 0$) drawn at the endpoint of the endoscopic instrument (see Figure 3.4) are shown here. As it is evident from Figure 3.5, the force feedback error will be limited ($\eta < 10 - 15\%$) if $\delta < 3°$. Therefore, a holding mechanism was devised in the haptic interface to place the PHANTOM in its zero position upon restart to ensure a small δ.

3.3.2 Workspace

In the haptic interface discussed in this chapter, we would like the endoscopic instrument to be horizontal at the reset position (which needs to be coincident with the PHANToM's home position to minimize force reflection errors) with its endpoint sweeping the space below as it starts to reach out to the intended body part. For this purpose, it is better to orient the PHANToM upside down. For the configuration in Figure 3.1, the workspace for the instrument covers a pitch angle of $\pm 30°$ (elbow up and down), a yaw angle of $\pm 40°$ (elbow left and right), a roll angle of $\pm 180°$ (rotation about the instrument axis) and an insertion depth of ± 11 cm (displacement along the instrument axis). Also, the gripping angle ranges from 0 to $30°$ (handle open and shut). On the other hand, for generic surgical tasks such as tissue handling, tissue dissection and suturing performed in-vivo by a number of surgeons in a minimally invasive environment, in 95% of the time the instruments have been found to be inside a $60°$ cone whose tip is located at the fulcrum [84]. Therefore, the workspace of the haptic user interface

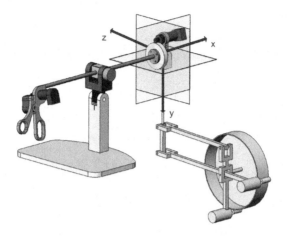

Fig. 3.4 The haptic interface and the $x = 0$, $y = 0$ and $z = 0$ planes at the instrument endpoint. Only a simplified view of the PHANToM device is shown.

does encompass the space typically reached by endoscopic instruments. As discussed in the next section, the PHANToM's orientation can be optimally selected based on the conditioning of the Jacobian matrix of the device.

3.3.2.1 *Optimization for control accuracy*

The control of a haptic device can be based on force control, position control or a combination of both. To improve the control accuracy for a robot, the Jacobian matrix condition number $\kappa = \|J\|\|J^{-1}\|$ where $\|J_{n \times n}\| = \sqrt{\text{trace}(JJ^{\text{T}}/n)}$ needs to be kept as small as possible at all points in the workspace. The condition number $1 < \kappa < \infty$ is a measure of the Jacobian invertibility (non-invertible for $\kappa = \infty$) and determines the accuracy of (a) the end effector force calculated from joint torque measurements that is essential for robot force control[3], and (b) the end effector Cartesian velocity calculated from joint angular velocity measurements that is essential for robot position control[4].

The global conditioning index (GCI) introduced in [44] determines the overall conditioning of the manipulator across the workspace W rather than

---

[3]Note that in open-loop force control, $F = (J^{\text{T}})^{-1}\tau_{\text{control}}$ governs the robot while in closed-loop force control, $F_{\text{measured}} = (J^{\text{T}})^{-1}\tau_{\text{measured}}$ is the feedback term.

[4]Note that in open-loop and closed-loop position control, $\dot{\theta}_{\text{control}} = (J^{\text{T}})^{-1}\dot{X}_{\text{desired}}$ and $\dot{\theta}_{\text{control}} = (J^{\text{T}})^{-1}(\dot{X}_{\text{desired}} - J\dot{\theta}_{\text{measured}})$ are the controllers, respectively.

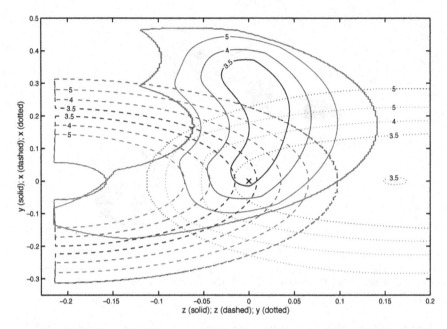

Fig. 3.5   Maximum normalized force feedback error (η) percentage per $1°$ angle offset (δ) at each point within the workspace: $x = 0$ plane (solid), $y = 0$ plane (dashed) and $z = 0$ plane (dotted) – the distances are in meters.

at each point therein:

$$\text{GCI} = \frac{\int_W (\frac{1}{\kappa}) \text{dW}}{\int_W \text{dW}} \tag{3.7}$$

Using the change of variable theorem[5], (3.7) can be written in the joint space as

$$\text{GCI} = \frac{\int_\Theta (\frac{1}{\kappa}) \det(J) \text{d}\theta_n \dots \text{d}\theta_1}{\int_\Theta \det(J) \text{d}\theta_n \dots \text{d}\theta_1} \tag{3.8}$$

Larger values of GCI correspond to better conditioning. The above index has previously been maximized over the space of the manipulator kinematic

---

[5]If x, y and z are functions of θ_1, θ_2 and θ_3, then

$$\int_{x,y,z} f(x,y,z) \text{d}x \text{d}y \text{d}z = \int_{\theta_1,\theta_2,\theta_3} f(x(\theta_1,\theta_2,\theta_3), y(\theta_1,\theta_2,\theta_3), z(\theta_1,\theta_2,\theta_3))$$

$$\det\left(\frac{\partial(x,y,z)}{\partial(\theta_1,\theta_2,\theta_3)}\right) \text{d}\theta_1 \text{d}\theta_2 \text{d}\theta_3.$$

Table 3.2   GCIs for two orientations of the PHANToM.

PHANToM orientation	Workspace boundaries	$\ell_2/\ell_1 = 0.79$	$\ell_2/\ell_1 = 0.96$
Normal	$\theta_2 \in (-55°, 90°)$ $\theta_3 \in (-40°, 90°)$	0.7679	0.7770
Upside down	$\theta_2 \in (0°, 90°)$ $\theta_3 \in (-40°, 90°)$	0.8154	0.8309

parameters [44]. We propose to use the GCI as a quantitative measure for optimal selection of the PHANToM's workspace, thereby determining which of the two orientations for the PHANToM favor the accuracy of control.

Table 3.2 compares the GCI's for the normal and upside-down orientations of the PHANToM. As can be seen, the GCI is higher for the upside-down orientation of the PHANToM where the desired motions of the endoscopic instrument exclude $\theta_2 \in (-55°, 0)$ from the PHANToM's workspace[6]. Therefore, for this particular application, it is even better for control purposes to orient the PHANToM in an upside-down configuration. Table 3.2 also shows that the additional attachment used to connect the PHANToM's endpoint to the instrument endpoint (thus increasing the second arm length and the ratio ℓ_2/ℓ_1) only helps to give a better conditioning index. This is because, as illustrated in Figures 3.6a and b, the GCI for the PHANToM takes its maximum value at $\theta_{2_{\min}} = 0$, $\theta_{3_{\min}} = 0$ and $\ell_2/\ell_1 = 1$ which is closest to the case when the PHANToM is upside down and the attachment exists.

The manipulability index $\mu = \sigma_{\min}(J)/\sigma_{\max}(J)$ of the haptic interface for the nominal values of the system parameters ($d = L/2$ and $\beta = 0$) is shown in Figure 3.7. As can be seen, this index is almost uniform in the neighborhood of the origin where the device is operated. Also note that the workspace is singularity free.

3.3.3   *Force reflection capability*

In line with the design specification of Section 3.2 regarding the force feedback range, we would like to determine the maximum magnitude of forces that the haptic interface is able to apply against the user's hand using a limited amount of torque. The motor torques τ and the end-

---

[6]Note that the integrands in the numerator and denominator of (3.8) are independent of θ_1. Also, the PHANToM's inverse kinematics relationships (C.2)-(C.4) in Appendix C were used in determining the workspace boundaries in terms of θ_2 and θ_3. In computing (3.8), the constraint on how close or apart the PHANToM's motors can get needs to be considered: $-50° < \theta_3 - \theta_2 < 50°$.

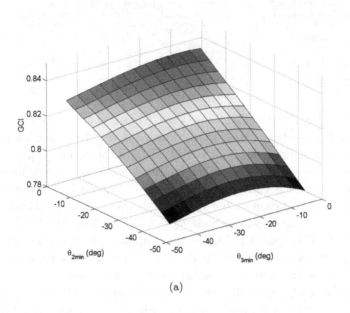

(a)

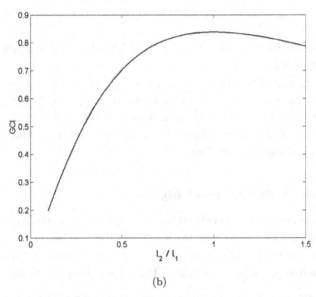

(b)

Fig. 3.6 (a) GCI versus $\theta_{2\min}$ and $\theta_{3\min}$ (the lower bounds of the integrals on θ_2 and θ_3) when the integral upper bounds are $\theta_{2\max} = \theta_{3\max} = 90°$ and $\ell_2/\ell_1 = 0.96$, and (b) GCI versus ℓ_2/ℓ_1 when $\theta_{2\min} = \theta_{3\min} = 0$ and $\theta_{2\max} = \theta_{3\max} = 90°$.

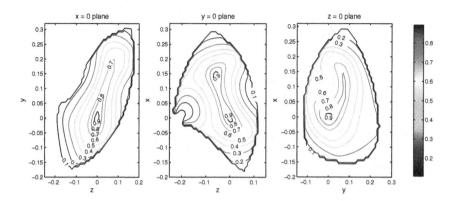

Fig. 3.7 Manipulability of the haptic interface at each point in the workspace – the distances are in meters.

point forces F of a robot are related through the Jacobian matrix as $F = (J^{\mathrm{T}}(\Theta))^{-1}\tau \doteq J_f(\Theta)\tau$. Therefore, for a unit torque vector ($\|\tau\|_2 = 1$), the limits on the magnitude of F are as follows by Theorem 3.1:

$$\sigma_{\min}(J_f) \le \|F\|_2 \le \sigma_{\max}(J_f) \tag{3.9}$$

For the haptic interface discussed in this chapter, using the Jacobian $J(\Theta, d, \beta, L)$ for the nominal system parameters ($d = L/2$ and $\beta = 0$), the iso-value contours of the maximum force that can be exerted on the user's hand using a unit torque vector are shown in Figure 3.8. With the unit torque assumption, the lower bound on the maximum force is 5 N across the workspace. For the PHANToM, in which the stall torque[7] of each motor is 240×10^{-3} Nm and the capstan drive's transmission ratio is 11.6:1, the actual maximum torque is $\|\tau\|_2 = 2.8\sqrt{3}$ Nm, meaning that the actual maximum force in each direction (F_x, F_y and F_z) is about 2.8 times larger than what is shown in Figure 3.8. For the gripping and roll directions of the haptic interface, equation (3.1) gives the maximum exertable forces to be 17 N and 12 N, respectively. Therefore, in all five degrees of freedom, the haptic interface meets our requirement on large force reflection, which is necessary for generating the high-stiffness response to emulate tool contact with a hard object such as bone.

---

[7]At maximum force (high stiffness resistance against the user's hand), the motor is almost steady.

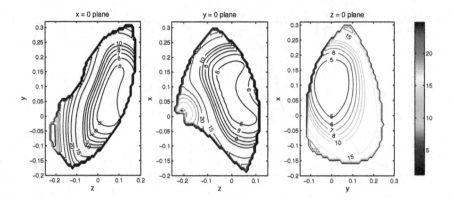

Fig. 3.8   Maximum force feedback for a unit torque at each point within the workspace
– the distances are in meters and forces are in Newtons.

3.4   Concluding Remarks

In this chapter, the need for haptic feedback in computer-integrated systems for endoscopic surgery and training was discussed. A haptic user interface suitable for endoscopic surgery was presented that can be used as part of a master-slave surgical teleoperator or in a virtual-reality surgical training system. Methods were proposed to analyze the characteristics of a haptic interface with regard to the sensitivity of force feedback to positioning errors, and the range of applicable end-point forces in relationship to the joint torques. Moreover, the workspace of the haptic interface was optimized for higher control accuracy. For more information about the master haptic interface discussed in this chapter, see Appendix B.

Chapter 4

Unilateral Teleoperation Control

4.1 Introduction

In unilateral master-slave teleoperation control, usually a fixed (PD or PID) controller is used to ensure convergence of the slave position to the master position provided the effects of gravity, friction, and Coriolis and centrifugal forces are pre-compensated using the knowledge of the slave dynamics. Using fixed position controllers is also common in bilateral teleoperation control such as the general bilateral control formalism proposed by Yokokohji et al. [153]. In this case, too, the dynamics of the master and the slave need to be known and fixed. In fact, with Yokokohji's bilateral controller, it can be shown that the singular values of the scattering matrix of the corresponding teleoperation system are equal to 1, implying that the teleoperation system passivity critically depends on having the exact dynamics of the master and the slave (see Theorem 5.4).

The PHANToM haptic device is commonly used as the master in haptics-based teleoperation research. Due to its ease of use and low friction, it is also used as the slave, e.g., in [104]. Whether used as the master or the slave, the PHANToM is a low inertia robot whose dynamics can vary significantly depending on the configuration (e.g. mounted on a wall, upside-down, or normally), the presence/absence of counterbalance weights and gimbal, and if a sensor or tool is attached at its endpoint. For control purposes, the dynamic model of the PHANToM can be identified for each particular model and configuration of the device and sensor/tool attachment [132], but this method is cumbersome and time consuming. Moreover, if used as part of a larger system, the PHANToM has to be mechanically separated from the rest of the system before its dynamic model parameters can be identified.

As a result, while the use of fixed position controllers may be justified for linear 1-DOF systems, we propose to use an adaptive scheme for trajectory control of the PHANToM robot. As suggested in [21], for a robot used as the slave in teleoperation tasks, an adaptive controller is needed to preserve master-slave position tracking when the environment impedance changes. As adaptive controllers, neural networks have been applied successfully in the identification and control of dynamic systems [38]. The universal approximation capabilities of the multi-layer perceptron make it a good choice for modeling nonlinear systems and for implementing nonlinear controllers. As an adaptive scheme, the learning capabilities of neural network controllers help them to cope with varying dynamic behaviors and operating conditions of a system.

Tracking based on *inverse dynamics control* has been the main thrust of research on neural networks for feedback control [17]. In inverse dynamics control, a neural network learns the inverse dynamics of a system provided the inverse model exists. This neural network can be trained off-line or on-line or a combination of both, as discussed below.

4.1.1   *Direct inverse dynamics control*

In direct inverse dynamics control, as shown in Figure 4.1a, the neural network learns during online feed-forward control. The network is trained to find the plant input that drives the system output to the reference value. The weights of the network are adjusted so that the error between the actual system output and the reference value is minimized in every iteration step. The problem of direct inverse dynamics control is that since the neural network in the only controller in the loop, the closed-loop system may become unstable at the first stages of learning. Therefore, it is necessary to provide initial estimates of the weights for the neural network, which may be acquired by prior off-line learning, in order to avoid instability.

4.1.2   *Feedback error learning control*

In the feedback error learning method, the neural network is used as a feed-forward controller which takes the desired trajectory as the input and is trained by using the output of a stabilizing feedback controller as the error signal (Figure 4.1b). As the neural network training progresses, the input error to the neural network diminishes, resulting in a greater contribution from the neural network controller to the feedback control. With

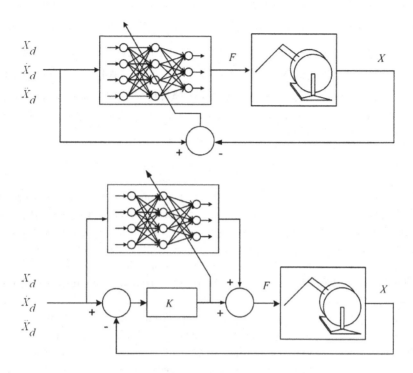

Fig. 4.1 (a) Direct inverse dynamics control (top), and (b) feedback error learning control (bottom).

this architecture, it is possible to start with a stable closed-loop system, even if the neural network has not been adequately trained.

4.2 PHANToM Inverse Dynamics Identification

The neural network controller used in either of the above-mentioned control methods is aimed at representing the inverse dynamics of the PHANToM, provided the inverse exists. Therefore, we first need to show that the inverse dynamics model of the PHANToM exists. The PHANToM dynamics can be written as [19]:

$$M(\theta)\ddot{\theta} + C(\theta, \dot{\theta})\dot{\theta} + N(\theta) = \tau \qquad (4.1)$$

where τ is the 3×1 vector of motor torques and θ is the 3×1 vector of joint angles. If $X = \begin{pmatrix} x & y & z \end{pmatrix}^{\mathrm{T}}$ is the endpoint Cartesian position and J is the Jacobian matrix, then $\dot{X} = J\dot{\theta}$ and $\ddot{X} = J\ddot{\theta} + \dot{J}\dot{\theta} = JM^{-1}(\tau - C\dot{\theta} -$

$N) + \dot{J}J^{-1}\dot{X}$. Now if we choose

$$\tau = MJ^{-1}(u - \dot{J}J^{-1}\dot{X}) + C\dot{\theta} + N \qquad (4.2)$$

$$u = \ddot{X}_r + K_d(\dot{X}_r - \dot{X}) + K_p(X_r - X) \qquad (4.3)$$

where X_r is the desired position of the PHANToM's endpoint, it is easy to see that the error e between the desired and the actual endpoint positions can be made to approach zero asymptotically through proper selection of the gains K_p and K_d:

$$\ddot{e} + K_d\dot{e} + K_p e = 0 \qquad (4.4)$$

Therefore, it is possible to use equations (4.2) and (4.3) to generate torques that drive the PHANToM governed by equation (4.1) to any desired position. This means that the inverse dynamics of the PHANToM exists. Indeed, equations (4.2) and (4.3) suggest a controller structure, which takes as input the desired and actual positions and velocities and desired accelerations and produces appropriate input torques to ensure asymptotic tracking.

For a neural network to learn the inverse dynamics of a system, first an input u is selected and applied to the system to obtain an output y, and then the neural network is trained to reproduce u at its output from y at its input. Figure 4.2 shows how a neural network is trained to represent the inverse dynamics of the PHANToM. Inspired by equations (4.2) and (4.3), the network has six position/velocity inputs $(x, \dot{x}, y, \dot{y}, z, \dot{z})$ and three force outputs (f_x, f_y, f_z). A two-layer back-propagation neural network with respectively six and three neurons in the hidden and the output layers is used. The activation function for the hidden layer is a bipolar sigmoid function

$$f(x) = \frac{1 - e^{-x}}{1 + e^{-x}} \qquad (4.5)$$

and that of the output layer is a linear function with saturation limits used to restrict the maximum output force as a safety precaution.

Two PHANToM 1.5A devices are used as the master and the slave. The real-time unilateral control of the slave PHANToM is implemented in a C++ environment. The neural network was trained offline by input/output data collected through an experiment in which arbitrary maneuvers were applied to the master by the user and the slave PHANToM was made to follow it via closed-loop control (proportional controller $K = 0.6$). The trained weights of the neural network were logged for use during real-time trajectory control of the slave PHANToM.

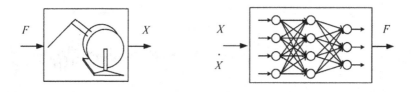

Fig. 4.2 Inverse dynamics model identification of the PHANToM robot.

4.3 Adaptive Inverse Dynamics Trajectory Control of the PHANToM

Having identified a fairly accurate inverse dynamics model of the system, we use it as the feed-forward controller in the feedback error learning method (Figure 4.1b). A proportional controller ($K = 0.6$) was used to stabilize the closed-loop system. The previously trained weights proved to be very helpful in stabilization in the first stage of learning. Third-order low-pass Butterworth filters were used on the master and slave position readings to avoid training the neural network by a fluctuating error signal. While the feedback control loop operates at 1 KHz, training was done once in five sampling times. In each training step, the back-propagation method performs steepest descent on the weight space to minimize the sum of error squares E. Therefore, the weights between hidden and output layers and those between input and hidden layers are adjusted according to

$$\Delta W_{ji} \propto -\frac{\partial E}{\partial W_{ji}} \qquad (4.6)$$

resulting in the following update laws:

$$W_{ji}(t+1) = W_{ji}(t) + \Delta W_{ji} \qquad (4.7)$$

$$\Delta W_{ji} = \eta \delta_j O_i \qquad (4.8)$$

For each layer, W_{ji} is the weight from unit i of the previous layer to the unit j in the current layer. O_i is the output of unit i of the previous layer, η is a gain called the learning rate, and δ_j is calculated differently for the hidden and output layers:

$$\text{Output} \quad \text{layer}: \quad \delta_j = (T_j - O_j)f'_j(S_j) \qquad (4.9)$$

$$\text{Hidden} \quad \text{layer}: \quad \delta_j = f'_j(S_j) \sum_k \delta_k W_{kj} \qquad (4.10)$$

Here,

$$S_j = \sum_i W_{ji} O_i \qquad (4.11)$$

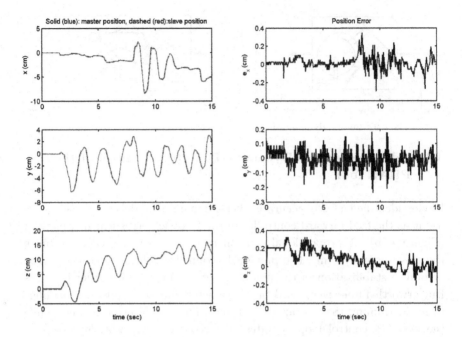

Fig. 4.3   Master and slave positions in feedback error learning control.

and T_j is the target value of the output of unit j. For each layer, while $\sum_k \delta_k W_{kj}$ is calculated over the next layer, S_j is calculated over the previous layer, and both use the weights of iteration $t-1$.

Figure 4.3 shows the results of an experiment in which the master underwent arbitrary hand movements and the slave manages to track it quite well. Moreover, the initial-guess weights of the neural network found by offline training prove to represent an accurate estimation of the system inverse dynamics because the weights remain in the ±5% vicinity of the initial values during on-line learning.

In another experiment, an additional mass (100 grams) was attached to the endpoint of the slave PHANToM to investigate the effect of an external disturbance (e.g. the unknown force vector due to a sensor). This affects the inertia matrix, the total mass, and the center of mass of the last link and hence the dynamics of the robot. A fixed MIMO control scheme such as computed torque control has the disadvantage that disturbances leave an undesirable steady-state tracking error, let alone the controller's dependence on perfect knowledge of the manipulator dynamics. However, as shown in Figures 4.4a, the tracking error is asymptotically reduced to zero with the feedback error learning control thanks to the online adaptability of the neural controller. The effect of the additional mass is neutralized by significant adaptation of the neural weights, particularly those associated with the output layer's second unit corresponding to the vertical component of the force vector (f_y), for example the weight W_{22} as shown in Figure 4.4b. This weight has ultimately reached a steady state because the disturbance is constant.

The training of a neural network controller can be stopped when the dynamics are satisfactorily captured. If the device is operated as the master or the slave during force-reflective teleoperation, hand/master and slave/environment interactions will occur. Obviously, changes in the dynamics that are caused by such interactions should not be included in the PHANToM dynamics; rather such information should be reflected to the user in the form of contact forces.

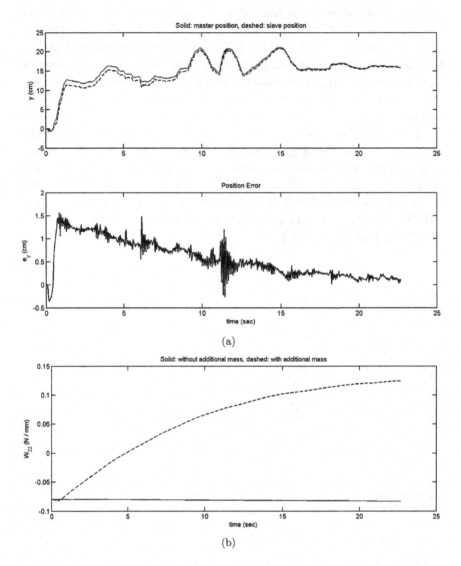

Fig. 4.4 From top to bottom: (a) Master and slave positions and position error in feedback error learning control in the presence of a disturbance, and (b) adaptation of a weight from the hidden layer to the output layer's f_y unit with and without the additional mass.

Chapter 5

Bilateral Teleoperation Control

5.1 Introduction

In master-slave teleoperation using a force-reflective human-machine interface (HMI), it is possible to reflect slave/environment interaction forces to
the user's hand merely based on the difference between the master and the
slave positions and without measurement of the slave/environment or the
hand/master contact forces. However, compared to such a "position error
based" method, the fidelity and reliability of haptic teleoperation can be
enhanced if the bilateral controller is fed with the measurements of master-
side and/or slave-side force sensors. Therefore, the issue that is addressed
in this chapter is the extent of benefits added by one or more force sensors and the effects of bilateral control structure on teleoperation stability
and transparency, which can be compromised due to implementation issues
and changes in the environment dynamics. We also study the effect of local
force feedback loops in terms of improving the robustness of teleoperation
system stability and performance. In the experiments in Section 5.3, which
are performed using a haptics-enabled master-slave testbed developed in
our lab, we compare the performance of two-channel and the four-channel
bilateral control architectures during soft-tissue palpation tests and explore
the role of local force feedback terms.

5.2 Stability and Transparency in Haptic Teleoperation

For safe and precise teleoperation, stability and transparency of the master-
slave system are essential. As a performance measure, Lawrence [79] has
defined transparency as "the description of the degree of telepresence of
the remote site available to the human operator through the teleoperator

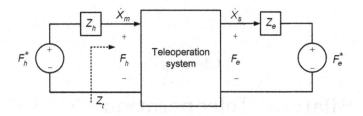

Fig. 5.1   Equivalent circuit representation of a teleoperation system.

device". Transparency of a bilaterally controlled teleoperator depends on how well the slave/environment interaction forces are reflected to the user's hand by the master. Denoting the hand/master interaction as f_h and the slave/environment interaction as f_e, the dynamics of the master and the slave can be written as:

$$f_m + f_h = M_m \ddot{x}_m, \quad f_s - f_e = M_s \ddot{x}_s \tag{5.1}$$

where M_m, M_s, x_m, x_s, f_m and f_s are the master and the slave inertias, positions and control signals (force or torque), respectively. In an ideally transparent teleoperation system, through appropriate control signals f_m and f_s, the master and the slave positions and interactions will match regardless of the operator and environment dynamics:

$$x_m = x_s, \quad f_h = f_e \tag{5.2}$$

By considering velocities and forces in a teleoperation system as currents and voltages, an equivalent circuit representation of the system can be obtained [48] (Figure 5.1), in which impedances $Z_h(s)$ and $Z_e(s)$ denote dynamic characteristics of the human operator's hand and the remote environment, respectively. Here, F_h^* and F_e^* are respectively the operator's and the environment's exogenous input forces and are independent of teleoperation system behavior. It is generally assumed that the environment is passive ($F_e^* = 0$) and the operator is passive in the sense that he/she does not perform actions that will make the teleoperation system unstable.

To evaluate the transparency of teleoperation, the hybrid representation of the two-port network model of a master-slave system is most suitable. In this representation:

$$\begin{bmatrix} F_h \\ -\dot{X}_s \end{bmatrix} = \begin{bmatrix} h_{11} & h_{12} \\ h_{21} & h_{22} \end{bmatrix} \cdot \begin{bmatrix} \dot{X}_m \\ F_e \end{bmatrix} \tag{5.3}$$

Note that we have used velocities in the hybrid representation rather than positions. This convention does not affect stability and transparency, although it might possibly cause small offsets between master and slave positions (steady-state errors in positions or position drifts) [79]. From (5.2) and (5.3), perfect transparency is achieved if and only if the hybrid matrix has the following form

$$H_{\text{ideal}} = \begin{bmatrix} 0 & 1 \\ -1 & 0 \end{bmatrix} \tag{5.4}$$

Each element of the H matrix has a physical meaning. The hybrid parameter $h_{11} = F_h/\dot{X}_m|_{F_e=0}$ is the input impedance in free-motion condition. Nonzero values for h_{11} mean that even when the slave is in free space, the user will receive some force feedback, thus giving a "sticky" feel of free-motion movements. The parameter $h_{12} = F_h/F_e|_{\dot{X}_m=0}$ is a measure of force tracking for the haptic teleoperation system when the master is locked in motion (perfect force tracking for $h_{12} = 1$). The parameter $h_{21} = -\dot{X}_s/\dot{X}_m|_{F_e=0}$ is a measure of position (velocity) tracking performance when the slave is in free space (perfect position/velocity tracking for $h_{21} = -1$). The parameter $h_{22} = -\dot{X}_s/F_e|_{\dot{X}_m=0}$ is the output admittance when the master is locked in motion. Nonzero values for h_{22} indicate that even when the master is locked in place, the slave will move in response to slave/environment contacts.

For analysis of stability of a teleoperation system, according to Figure 5.1, the knowledge of the human operator and the environment dynamics are needed in addition to the teleoperation system model (5.3). However, assuming that $Z_h(s)$ and $Z_e(s)$ are passive, we might be able to draw stability conditions independent of the human operator and the environment (*absolute stability*). The necessary and sufficient conditions for absolute stability (stability under all passive terminations $Z_h(s)$ and $Z_e(s)$) of a two-port network are given by the following theorem [53]:

Theorem 5.1 (Llewellyn's criterion). *The teleoperation system (5.3) is absolutely stable if and only if: (a) $h_{11}(s)$ and $h_{22}(s)$ have no poles in the right half plane (RHP); (b) any poles of $h_{11}(s)$ and $h_{22}(s)$ on the imaginary axis are simple with real and positive residues; and (c) for $s = j\omega$ and all real values of ω*

$$\Re(h_{11}) \geq 0 \tag{5.5}$$

$$\Re(h_{22}) \geq 0 \tag{5.6}$$

$$2\Re(h_{11})\Re(h_{22}) - \Re(h_{12}h_{21}) - |h_{12}h_{21}| \geq 0 \tag{5.7}$$

where $\Re(\cdot)$ and $|\cdot|$ denote the real and absolute values. $\Diamond$

For achieving the ideal response (5.4), various teleoperation control architectures are proposed in the literature. These control architectures are usually classified as position-force (i.e. position control at the master side and force control at the slave side), force-position, position-position, and force-force architectures. Among these four architectures, in order to have a stiff slave, we are interested in those in which the slave is under position control, namely position-position and force-position. A more general classification is by the number of communication channels required for transmitting position and force values from the master to the slave and vice versa in each bilateral control architecture. In the following, we discuss the stability and transparency of the above-mentioned two-channel architectures in addition to a more sophisticated four-channel architecture.

5.2.1   *2-channel architectures*

5.2.1.1   *Position Error Based (PEB)*

A position-error based, also called position-position, teleoperation architecture is shown in Figure 5.2a. The impedances $Z_m(s) = M_m s$ and $Z_s(s) = M_s s$ represent the dynamic characteristics of the master robot and the slave robot, respectively. Also, $C_m = (k_{v_m} s + k_{p_m})/s$ and $C_s = (k_{v_s} s + k_{p_s})/s$ are proportional-derivative controllers used at the master and the slave, respectively (here the master and the slave velocities are fed to the two controllers).

As can be seen in Figure 5.2a, the PEB controller does not use any force sensor measurements (no shaded block with a force input) and merely tries to minimize the difference between the master and the slave positions, thus reflecting a force proportional to this difference to the user once the slave makes contact with an object. The hybrid matrix for this architecture is given as

$$H = \begin{bmatrix} Z_m + C_m \frac{Z_s}{Z_{ts}} & \frac{C_m}{Z_{ts}} \\ -\frac{C_s}{Z_{ts}} & \frac{1}{Z_{ts}} \end{bmatrix} \tag{5.8}$$

where $Z_{tm} = Z_m + C_m$, $Z_{ts} = Z_s + C_s$. As a result, in addition to non-ideal force tracking ($h_{12} \neq 1$), the PEB method suffers from a distorted perception in free-motion condition ($h_{11} \neq 0$). This means that in the absence of a slave-side force sensor, control inaccuracies (i.e., nonzero position

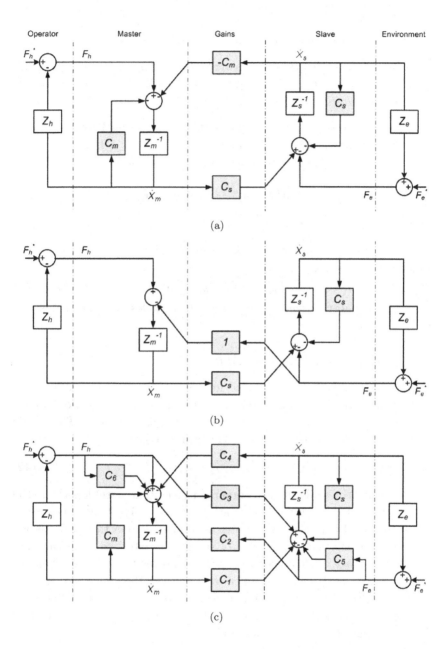

Fig. 5.2 (a) Position-error based, (b) direct force reflection, and (c) 4-channel bilateral control architectures. The shaded blocks represent control components.

errors) lead to proportional force feedback to the user even when the slave is not in contact with the environment.

Theorem 5.2. *The position error based teleoperation system of Figure 5.2a is absolutely stable if $k_{v_m}, k_{p_m}, k_{v_s}, k_{p_s} > 0$ and $C_m(s)/C_s(s) = \alpha$ where α is a positive constant.*

Proof. To investigate the stability of this system using Theorem 5.1, the characteristic polynomial for h_{11} and h_{22} is $M_s s^2 + k_{v_s} s + k_{p_s}$, which has no RHP poles if $k_{v_s}, k_{p_s} > 0$. With respect to conditions (5.5) and (5.6), we have

$$\Re(h_{11}) = \frac{M_s(k_{v_s} k_{p_m} - k_{v_m} k_{p_s} + M_s k_{v_m} \omega^2)}{k_{v_s}^2 + (-k_{p_s}/\omega + M_s \omega)^2} \tag{5.9}$$

$$\Re(h_{22}) = \frac{k_{v_s}}{k_{v_s}^2 + (-k_{p_s}/\omega + M_s \omega)^2} \tag{5.10}$$

which are non-negative if $k_{v_m} > 0$, $k_{v_s} > 0$ and

$$k_{v_s} k_{p_m} - k_{v_m} k_{p_s} = 0 \tag{5.11}$$

Also, the equality to zero in condition (5.7) holds if (5.11) holds and $k_{v_m}, k_{p_m} > 0$. □

5.2.1.2 Direct Force Reflection (DFR)

A direct force reflection, also called force-position, teleoperation architecture is shown in Figure 5.2b. This method requires a force sensor to measure the interactions between the slave and the environment. The hybrid parameters for the force-position architecture are given as

$$H = \begin{bmatrix} Z_m & 1 \\ -\dfrac{C_s}{Z_{ts}} & \dfrac{1}{Z_{ts}} \end{bmatrix} \tag{5.12}$$

Consequently, while the perception of free-motion is still less than ideal ($h_{11} \neq 0$), perfect force tracking is attained ($h_{12} = 1$). Nonetheless, compared to the PEB method, h_{11} is much closer to zero in the DFR method and the user only feels the inertia of the master interface when the slave is not in contact. While the DFR method proves to be better than the PEB method, both methods suffer from the less-than-ideal h_{21} and h_{22} values, resulting in poor position tracking response and slave stiffness. In Section 5.2.2, we will explain how a 4-channel architecture can fulfil all of the conditions of the ideal response (5.4).

Theorem 5.3. *The direct force reflection teleoperation system of Figure 5.2b is absolutely stable if $k_{v_s}, k_{p_s} > 0$ and $|C_s| \gg |Z_s|$.*

Proof. To investigate the stability via Theorem 5.1, h_{11} has no poles and the characteristic polynomial for h_{22} is $M_s s^2 + k_{v_s} s + k_{p_s}$, which has no RHP poles if $k_{v_s}, k_{p_s} > 0$. Also, $\Re(h_{11}) = 0$ and $\Re(h_{22})$ is same as (5.10), which is non-negative if $k_{v_s} > 0$. Also, condition (5.7) is simplified to

$$\Re\left(\frac{C_s}{C_s + Z_s}\right) - \left|\frac{C_s}{C_s + Z_s}\right| \geq 0 \tag{5.13}$$

Equation (5.13) holds if and only if

$$\Im\left(\frac{C_s}{C_s + Z_s}\right) = \frac{k_{v_s}\omega M_s}{k_{v_s}^2 + (-k_{p_s}/\omega + M_s\omega)^2} = 0 \tag{5.14}$$

which is mathematically true provided $k_{v_s} = 0$, i.e., no derivative term is used at the slave side, which is not a viable option. However, the imaginary part (5.14) approaches zero if $k_{p_s} \to \infty$, $k_{v_s} \to \infty$ or $M_s \to 0$, which can be summarized as $|C_s| \gg |Z_s|$. $\qquad\square$

Using a loop-shaping filter can help to achieve a higher degree of absolute stability [35]. Nevertheless, the above discussion is conservative as it ensures stability regardless of the teleoperation system's terminations. For a less conservative study, taking into account the remote environment impedance Z_e, i.e., $F_e = Z_e \dot{X}_s$, the general teleoperation system given by (5.3) has the following transfer function from F_h to $\dot{X}_m$:

$$\frac{\dot{X}_m}{F_h} = \frac{1 + h_{22}Z_e}{h_{11}(1 + h_{22}Z_e) - h_{12}h_{21}Z_e} \tag{5.15}$$

Assuming the environment is modeled by a linear spring, $Z_e = k_e/s$, the characteristic equation for the transfer function from F_h to $\dot{X}_m$ (and to any other output), which must have no zeros in the right-half plane (RHP) for the teleoperation system to be stable, is given by

$$h_{11}s + k_e(h_{11}h_{22} - h_{12}h_{21}) = 0 \tag{5.16}$$

Using the hybrid parameters (5.12) and $C_s = (k_{v_s}s + k_{p_s})/s$, (5.16) simplifies to

$$M_m M_s s^4 + M_m k_{v_s} s^3 + M_m(k_e + k_{p_s})s^2 + k_e k_{v_s} s + k_e k_{p_s} = 0 \tag{5.17}$$

Applying the Routh-Hurwitz criterion to (5.17), the necessary and sufficient conditions for asymptotic stability of the teleoperation system are

$$\Delta_1 = \frac{k_{v_s}}{M_s} > 0, \quad \Delta_2 = \frac{k_{v_s}[\beta k_{p_s} + k_e(\beta - 1)]}{M_s M_m} > 0$$

$$\Delta_3 = \frac{k_{v_s}^2 k_e^2(\beta - 1)}{M_s^2 M_m^2} > 0, \quad \Delta_4 = \frac{k_{v_s}^2 k_e^3 k_{p_s}(\beta - 1)}{M_s^3 M_m^3} > 0 \tag{5.18}$$

Table 5.1   The 4-channel architecture versus several simpler architectures.

Bilateral control method	C_1	C_2	C_3	C_4	C_5	C_6	C_m	C_s	no. chan.
Position-error based	$\checkmark$	-	-	$\checkmark$	-	-	$\checkmark$	$\checkmark$	2
Direct force reflection	$\checkmark$	$\checkmark$	-	-	-	-	-	$\checkmark$	2
Shared compliance	$\checkmark$	$\checkmark$	-	-	$\checkmark$	-	-	$\checkmark$	2
Bilateral impedance [82]	$\checkmark$	$\checkmark$	-	$\checkmark$	$\checkmark$	$\checkmark$	$\checkmark$	$\checkmark$	3

where $\beta = M_m/M_s$. The above condition set holds iff

$$k_{v_s} > 0, \quad k_{p_s} > 0, \quad \beta > 1 \tag{5.19}$$

While we have considered a unity force feedback gain in Figure 5.2b, if a gain $k_f \neq 1$ is used, the condition $\beta > 1$ is changed to $\beta > k_f$. The condition set (5.19) guarantees stability independent of frequency.

5.2.2   *4-channel architecture*

Figure 5.2c depicts a general 4-channel (4CH) bilateral teleoperation architecture [79, 153]. This architecture can represent other teleoperation structures through appropriate selection of subsystem dynamics C_1 to C_6 (see Table 5.1). The compensators C_5 and C_6 in Figure 5.2c constitute local force feedback at the slave side and the master side, respectively. The H-parameters for the 4CH architecture in Figure 5.2c are:

$$h_{11} = (Z_{ts}Z_{tm} + C_1C_4)/D$$
$$h_{12} = [Z_{ts}C_2 - (1 + C_5)C_4]/D$$
$$h_{21} = -[Z_{tm}C_3 + (1 + C_6)C_1]/D$$
$$h_{22} = -[C_2C_3 - (1 + C_5)(1 + C_6)]/D \tag{5.20}$$

where $D = -C_3C_4 + Z_{ts}(1 + C_6)$.

In contrast to the 2-channel (2CH) architectures, a sufficient number of parameters (degrees of freedom) in the 4CH architecture enables it to achieve ideal transparency. In fact, by selecting C_1 through C_6 according to

$$C_1 = Z_{ts}, \quad C_2 = 1 + C_6$$
$$C_3 = 1 + C_5, \quad C_4 = -Z_{tm} \tag{5.21}$$

the ideal transparency conditions (5.4) are fully met.

For analysis of stability, we need to use scattering theory, which is a powerful tool for investigation of absolute stability in two-port networks.

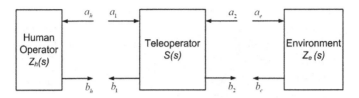

Fig. 5.3   A generalized description of a bilateral teleoperation system in terms of scattering parameters.

5.2.2.1   *Scattering theory and absolute stability*

According to Colgate [24]: *A bilateral teleoperation system is said to be robustly (or absolutely) stable if, when coupled to any passive environment, it presents to the operator an impedance (admittance) which is passive.* It is generally assumed that the human operator is passive, i.e., the operator does not perform actions to make the system unstable. Based on its scattering matrix model and according to Figure 5.3, a teleoperation system is represented as

$$b = S(s)a = \begin{bmatrix} S_{11}(s) & S_{12}(s) \\ S_{21}(s) & S_{22}(s) \end{bmatrix} a \tag{5.22}$$

Here, $a = [a_1 \ a_2]^T$ and $b = [b_1 \ b_2]^T$ are respectively the input and output waves of the teleoperation system, and are related to equivalent voltages and currents as:

$$a = (F + n^2\dot{X})/2, \quad b = (F - n^2\dot{X})/2 \tag{5.23}$$

where $F = [F_h \ F_e]^T$, $\dot{X} = [\dot{X}_m \ -\dot{X}_s]^T$, and n is a scaling factor. The following theorem gives a necessary and sufficient condition for absolute stability of a teleoperation system.

Theorem 5.4. *The necessary and sufficient condition for stability in a reciprocal two-port network ($S_{12} = S_{21}$) with an RHP-analytic scattering matrix $S(s)$ that is terminated with a passive operator and a passive environment is [24]:*

$$\bar{\sigma}[S(j\omega)] \le 1 \tag{5.24}$$

where $\bar{\sigma}$ represents the maximum singular value of $S(j\omega)$. In the case of a non-reciprocal two-port network, the passivity condition (5.24) in only a sufficient condition for stability[152, 24]. ◇

The smaller $\bar{\sigma}(S)$ is for a teleoperation system, the larger are the stability margin of the system and the stability robustness of the closed-loop system against variations in the dynamic parameters of the master, the slave and the controller.

The relation between the scattering matrix $S(s)$ and the hybrid matrix $H(s)$ of a two-port network is given by

$$S(s) = \begin{bmatrix} 1 & 0 \\ 0 & -1 \end{bmatrix} (H(s) - I)(H(s) + I)^{-1} \tag{5.25}$$

Theorem 5.5. *The necessary and sufficient condition for absolute stability of the 4CH teleoperation system of Figure 5.2c under ideal transparency conditions is that all coefficients of polynomial*

$$\begin{aligned} D &= C_3 Z_{tm} + C_2 Z_{ts} \\ &= (M_m C_3 + M_s C_2)s^2 + (k_{dm} C_3 + k_{ds} C_2)s \\ &\quad + k_{pm} C_3 + k_{ps} C_2 \end{aligned} \tag{5.26}$$

have the same sign.

Proof. In the 4CH architecture, when the ideal transparency condition set (5.21) holds, the hybrid matrix is

$$H = \begin{bmatrix} 0 & \frac{D}{D} \\ -\frac{D}{D} & 0 \end{bmatrix} \tag{5.27}$$

where D is found to be as given in (5.26) given that $Z_{tm} = M_m s + C_m(s) = M_m s + k_{dm} + k_{pm}/s$ and $Z_{ts} = M_s s + C_s(s) = M_s s + k_{ds} + k_{ps}/s$. The above hybrid matrix corresponds to the following scattering matrix:

$$S = \begin{bmatrix} \frac{-D^2 + D^2}{2D^2} & \frac{2D^2}{2D^2} \\ \frac{2D^2}{2D^2} & \frac{D^2 - D^2}{2D^2} \end{bmatrix} \tag{5.28}$$

For scattering matrix S in (5.28) to be RHP-analytic, D has to be Hurwitz. The necessary and sufficient condition for D being Hurwitz is that all the coefficients have the same sign. In this case, S can be simplified to

$$S = \begin{bmatrix} 0 & 1 \\ 1 & 0 \end{bmatrix} \tag{5.29}$$

Both of the singular values of this matrix are equal to 1. Therefore, since under ideal transparency condition the system is reciprocal, according to (5.24), the system is absolutely stable iff all the coefficients in the polynomial D given in (5.26) have the same sign. $\qquad\square$

5.2.2.2 *Stability and performance robustness*

It should be noted that under ideal transparent conditions, i.e., when the singular values of $S(s)$ are 1, the passivity (and stability) critically depends on exact implementation of control laws and having the exact dynamics of the master and the slave as any non-ideality might increase the maximum singular value beyond unity. Such a low stability margin can be explained by the trade-off that exists between stability and transparency in bilateral teleoperation [79, 72]. In the following, we study the effects of two control implementation issues on the teleoperation system stability and performance.

In practice, the ideal transparency conditions $C_1 = Z_{ts} = C_s + Z_s$ and $C_4 = -Z_{tm} = -C_m - Z_m$ are difficult to meet exactly due to the noise that would be introduced into the system by the acceleration terms. Therefore, approximations $C_1 = C_s + (\gamma + 1)Z_s$ and $C_4 = -C_m - (\gamma + 1)Z_m$ where $-1 \leq \gamma < 0$ are made, which affect the teleoperation transparency and more importantly, the stability of an already critically stable system. To examine the effect of $\gamma \neq 0$ on system stability, let us derive the characteristic polynomial for the transfer function $\dot{X}_m/F_h$:

$$M_m M_s(\gamma + 2)\gamma s^4 + (M_m k_{v_s} + M_s k_{v_m})\gamma s^3 + \qquad (5.30)$$
$$((M_s k_{p_m} + M_m k_{p_s} - k_e M_s(1 + C_6))\gamma -$$
$$(k_e M_m(1 + C_5) + k_e M_s(1 + C_6))s^2 -$$
$$(k_e k_{v_m}(1 + C_5) + k_e k_{v_s}(1 + C_6))s -$$
$$(k_e k_{p_m}(1 + C_5) + k_e k_{p_s}(1 + C_6)) = 0$$

Fortunately, when $\gamma \neq 0$, the presence of local force feedback terms C_5 and C_6 gives extra degrees of freedom to stabilize an otherwise unstable system. To further illustrate this point, consider $M_m = 5.968 \times 10^{-4}$ kgm^2 and $M_s = 9.814 \times 10^{-3}$ kgm^2. These values have been extracted from our experimental setup, which will be described in Section 5.3.1. Also, $C_m(s) = M_m(80s + 1600)/s$, $C_m(s) = M_s(80s + 1600)/s$, which position the master and the slave closed loop poles (in free motion) at $(-40, -40)$. Moreover, assume that the environment is modeled by a spring $Z_e = k_e/s$ where $k_e = 100$ N/m. If the acceleration terms are ignored in the control laws C_1 and C_4 (i.e., $\gamma = -1$), the absence of local force feedback terms $(C_5 = C_6 = 0)$ leads to a pair of RHP poles $(-280.3, -20.3, 70.3 \pm j212.2)$. However, as shown in Figure 5.4, introducing local force feedback terms, e.g., $C_5 > -1$ and $C_6 = -1$, can shift the unstable poles to stable locations.

In order to investigate the effect of local force feedback on transparency

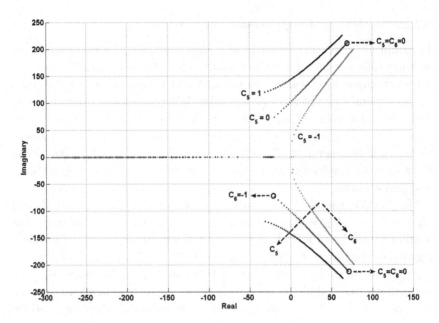

Fig. 5.4 Root loci of the poles of the 4CH teleoperation system with $\gamma = -1$ when $-1 \le C_6 \le 0$ and $C_5 = 1, 0, -1$.

when $\gamma \ne 0$, let us define the transparency transfer function of the general teleoperation system described by (5.3) as

$$T = \frac{Z_t}{Z_e} = \frac{h_{11} + (h_{11}h_{22} - h_{12}h_{21})Z_e}{(1 + h_{22}Z_e)Z_e} \tag{5.31}$$

where, as shown in Figure 5.1, Z_t is the impedance transmitted to and felt by the operator. Under ideal transparency and $\gamma = 0$, we have $T = 1$ regardless of the remote environment Z_e. However, $\gamma \ne 0$ makes T dependent on Z_e. To reduce the dependence of T on Z_e, let us define the transparency sensitivity function as

$$S_T = \frac{\partial T}{\partial Z_e} = \frac{\gamma[Z_m(C_s + \gamma Z_s) + Z_m(C_m + 2Z_m)]}{[(1 + C_5)(Z_{tm} + \gamma Z_m) + (1 + C_6)Z_{ts}]Z_e^2} \tag{5.32}$$

To see the effect of C_5 and C_6 on performance robustness, a sensitivity ratio is defined:

$$R = \frac{S_T|_{C_5 \ne 0, C_6 \ne 0}}{S_T|_{C_5 = C_6 = 0}}$$

$$= \frac{Z_m \gamma + Z_{tm} + Z_{ts}}{(1 + C_5)(Z_{tm} + \gamma Z_m) + (1 + C_6)Z_{ts}} \tag{5.33}$$

As can be seen, compared to the case of no local force feedback, the presence of local force feedback terms e.g., $C_6 = -1$ and sufficiently large $C_5 > 0$, can make $R < 1$, thus reducing the dependence of the transparency transfer function T on Z_e.

Local force feedback terms C_5 and C_6 also help mitigate the undesirable effects of processing delay and communication latency between the master and the slave. In the presence of time delay T_d, an ideally transparent bilateral teleoperation system has the hybrid matrix

$$H = \begin{bmatrix} 0 & e^{-sT_d} \\ -e^{-sT_d} & 0 \end{bmatrix} \qquad (5.34)$$

For this two-port network, the scattering matrix can be written as

$$S = \begin{bmatrix} -\tanh(sT_d) & \mathrm{sech}(sT_d) \\ \mathrm{sech}(sT_d) & \tanh(sT_d) \end{bmatrix} \qquad (5.35)$$

It can be shown that $\bar{\sigma}(S)$ for this scattering matrix is unbounded, consequently this system cannot maintain stability for all passive operators and environments. However, when Z_h and Z_e are factored in the analysis, the teleoperation system loses its reciprocity property and therefore, although not passive, it can be stabilized by proper choices of Z_h and Z_e [52].

According to (5.31), the hybrid matrix (5.34) corresponds to the following ideal transparency transfer function: $T = e^{-2sT_d}$. In the 4CH architecture under time delay, when the ideal transparency condition set (5.21) holds, the transparency transfer function is given by

$$T = \frac{Z_{tm}C_3 + Z_{ts}C_2 e^{-2sT_d} + Z_{tm}Z_{ts}/Z_e(1 - e^{-2sT_d})}{Z_e(1 - e^{-2sT_d})C_3C_2 + Z_{ts}C_2 + Z_{tm}e^{-2sT_d}C_3} \qquad (5.36)$$

It can be easily seen that in the absence of local force feedback terms ($C_6 = C_2 - 1 = 0, C_5 = C_3 - 1 = 0$), $T \neq e^{-2sT_d}$. However, with nonzero C_5 and C_6, near-ideal transparency can be achieved. For instance, taking $C_5 = -1$, (5.36) will be reduced to

$$T = e^{-2sT_d} + \frac{Z_{tm}}{Z_e C_2}(1 - e^{-2sT_d}) \qquad (5.37)$$

which approaches the ideal $T = e^{-2sT_d}$ by selecting a sufficiently large C_2. To further illustrate this point, Figure 5.5 shows the magnitude of the frequency response of the transparency transfer function T for the example described earlier with $C_5 = -1$ and one-way delays of $T_d = 15$ msec (top) and $T_d = 150$ msec (bottom). Evidently, with an increase in C_2, the magnitude of T nears 1 over a relatively wide frequency range.

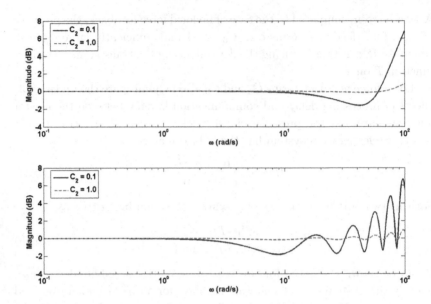

Fig. 5.5   The transparency transfer function magnitude for one-way delays $T_d = 15$ msec (top) and $T_d = 150$ msec (bottom).

5.2.2.3   *3-channel case*

Another potential benefit of the general 4CH architecture of Figure 5.2c is that by proper adjustment of the local feedback parameters, it is possible to obtain two classes of 3-channel (3CH) control architectures, which can be transparent under ideal conditions [52]. The first class of 3CH architectures is derived by setting $C_2 = 1$ and $C_3 = 0$. As a consequence, $C_5 = -1$ and $C_6 = 0$. In other words, there is no need for master/operator interaction force measurement and therefore, the number of sensors in the system can be reduced. The second class of 3CH architectures is obtained by setting $C_2 = 0$ and $C_3 = 1$. In this class, force measurement at the slave side is not needed. The need for fewer sensors without imposing additional expense on system transparency makes the 3CH architectures extremely attractive from the implementation point of view.

5.3   Haptic Teleoperation Experiments

5.3.1   *Experimental setup*

For experimental evaluation of the different haptic teleoperation control methods described in Section 5.2, we used the bilateral master-slave system consisting the master interface of Chapter 3 and the slave robot of Chapter 2. In Figure 5.6 and the experiments in this chapter, the master and slave subsystems were constrained for force-reflective teleoperation in the twist direction only (i.e. rotations about the instrument axis). The digital control loop was implemented at a sampling frequency of 1000 Hz. As discussed in Appendix D, the friction and gravity effects present in the master were determined and compensated for such that the user does not feel any weight on his/her hand when the slave is not in contact with an object. Appendix D also includes the master system modeling and identification, whereby the friction-compensated master is represented as $\tau_m = M_m \ddot{\theta}_m$ where $M_m = 5.97 \times 10^{-4}$ kgm^2. Using a similar method, the slave's model was identified as $\tau_s = M_s \ddot{\theta}_s$ where $M_s = 9.8 \times 10^{-3}$.

5.3.2   *Master-slave communication*

The Virtual Reality Peripheral Network (VRPN) has been used to establish network-based communication between the master and slave subsystems so that the slave can be telemanipulated by the user sitting at the master haptic interface possibly located at a distant location. VRPN provides a network-transparent and device-independent interface to virtual reality peripherals [138]. See Appendix E for a detailed description of the VRPN capabilities and how VRPN can be used in the context of master-slave teleoperation. In the following, communication between the master and the slave using VRPN is briefly discussed.

In the configuration shown in Figure 5.7, two PCs (P4, 2.8 GHz) called the master server and the slave server are placed local to the master and the slave, respectively. Through their I/O cards, these two PCs input (output) the measured variables (the control actions) from (to) the master and the slave. The measured variables are the master and slave positions x_h ($=x_m$) and x_e ($=x_s$) and forces f_h and f_e while the control actions are f_m and f_s. A third PC, which runs the algorithms for the master control and the slave control at the rate of 1 KHz, communicates in each sampling time through VRPN with the two local PCs for data exchange. Due to the proximity of

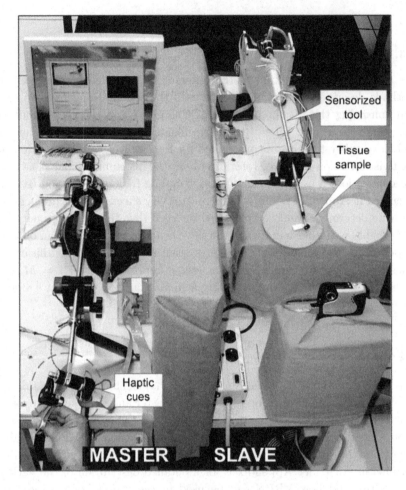

Fig. 5.6 Master-slave experimental setup.

different components of the master-slave system, in the experiments in this Chapter, the communication latency T_d is negligible.

5.3.3 *Observation of hand forces*

The 4CH bilateral control method requires the measurements of hand/master interactions f_h and slave/environment interactions f_e. In our master-slave system, while the slave's end-effector is sensorized to directly measure f_e, we need to use the dynamic model of the master to estimate f_h

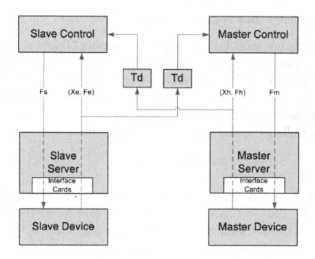

Fig. 5.7 Master-slave communication.

using a state observer. For this purpose, let us write the master dynamics $f_m + f_h = M_m \ddot{x}_m$ in state-space form by choosing $x_1 = x_m$ and $x_2 = \dot{x}_m$:

$$\dot{x}_1 = x_2$$
$$\dot{x}_2 = M_m^{-1}(f_m + f_h)$$

To estimate the hand force f_h (and the joint velocity $\dot{x}_m$), the Nicosia observer was used [100]:

$$\dot{\hat{x}}_1 = \hat{x}_2 + k_2 e$$
$$\dot{\hat{x}}_2 = M_m^{-1}(x_m + k_1 e)$$
$$e = x_1 - \hat{x}_1 \tag{5.38}$$

where k_1 and k_2 are positive constants. The observer uses the joint position and the portion of the joint torque that comes from the controller to find the externally applied joint torque. It can be shown that the observer is asymptotically stable and the error equation is:

$$M_m \ddot{e} + k_2 M_m \dot{e} + k_1 e = f_h \tag{5.39}$$

In steady state, $\ddot{e} = \dot{e} = 0$. Therefore, the hand force is estimated at low frequencies as $\bar{f}_h = k_1 e$.

5.3.4   *Observer and controller gains*

Using the dynamic model of the master (Appendix D) and in the absence of a force sensor at the master, the observer (5.38) was used to estimate the hand forces f_h. Using the observer's error dynamics (5.39), the gains k_1 and $k_2 = 2\sqrt{k_1/M_m}$ were chosen such that the observer has very fast, critically-damped poles at $(-350 \quad -350)$.

The controllers C_m and C_s should be chosen as

$$\frac{C_s}{C_m} = \frac{M_s}{M_m} \qquad (5.40)$$

as the master and the slave control actions need to be proportional to their inertias. This will ensure that the master and the slave have similar closed-loop behavior. Therefore, we take $C_m = M_m(k_v s + k_p)/s$ and $C_s = M_s(k_v s + k_p)/s$ noting that the master and the slave velocities are fed to the two controllers. To place the master and the slave closed-loop poles for fast responses, $(k_p \quad k_v) = (1600 \quad 80)$ were chosen. This results in the position error characteristic equation $\ddot{e}_x + 80\dot{e}_x + 1600 e_x = 0$ where $e_x = x_m - x_s$ for both the master and the slave (both in free space), thus moving the closed-loop poles of the master and the slave to $(-40 \quad -40)$.

5.3.5   *Soft-tissue palpation tests*

In a palpation test, the user twists the master back and forth causing the slave to repeatedly probe a soft tissue phantom using a small rigid beam attached to the slave's end-effector for 60 seconds. The user receives haptic feedback of instrument/tissue interactions in real-time. In addition to the above-mentioned tests and to further investigate the relative transparency of systems, a second set of free-motion tests are performed, which in conjunction with the previous contact-mode tests, can be used to determine the hybrid parameters of the teleoperation system in the frequency domain. In the free-motion tests, the master is moved back and forth by the user for about 60 seconds, while the slave's tip is in free space. Since $f_e = 0$, the frequency responses $h_{11} = F_h/X_m$ and $h_{21} = -X_s/X_m$ can be found by applying spectral analysis (MATLAB function *spa*) on the free-motion test data (for the two-port hybrid model based on positions rather than velocities). By using the contact-mode test data, the other two hybrid parameters can be obtained as $h_{12} = F_h/F_e - h_{11}X_m/F_e$ and $h_{22} = -X_s/F_e - h_{21}X_m/F_e$.

Figure 5.8 shows the master and the slave position and torque tracking

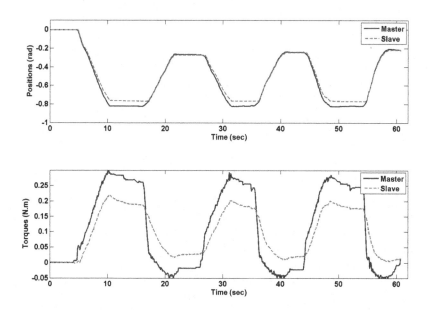

Fig. 5.8   Position and force profiles for the PEB teleoperation system.

profiles in the contact mode for the PEB teleoperation system. Figure 5.9 illustrates the same profiles for the DFR system. As can be seen, the DFR system displays a superior force tracking performance compared to PEB. The magnitudes of the hybrid parameters of the PEB and DFR teleoperation systems are shown in Figure 5.10. Due to the human operator's limited input bandwidth, these identified hybrid parameters can be considered valid up to a frequency of 60 rad/s.

Figure 5.10 is an indication of DFR's superiority in terms of transparent performance considering the ideal transparency requirement (5.4). As expected from equations (5.8) and (5.12), relatively high values of h_{11} for PEB are evidence of the fact that even when the slave is in free space, the user will feel some force, giving a "sticky" feel of free-motion movements. On the other hand, since DFR uses f_e measurements, its input impedance in free-motion condition (h_{11}) will be lower making the feel of free space much more realistic. The better force tracking performance of DFR, i.e., $h_{12} \approx 0$ dB, agrees with the time-domain plots of Figures 5.8 and 5.9 and, more importantly, confirms equation (5.12). With regard to h_{21}, both spectra are close to 0 dB, which indicates both systems ensure good position tracking in free space. These results are in accordance with equations (5.8)

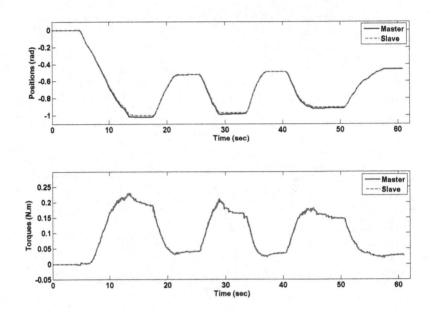

Fig. 5.9   Position and force profiles for the DFR teleoperation system.

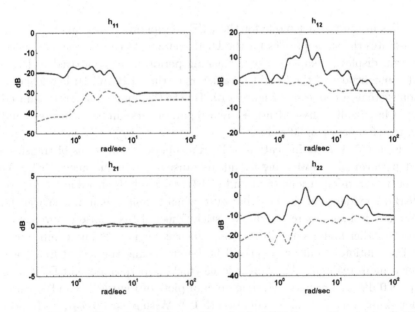

Fig. 5.10   Magnitudes of the hybrid parameters for the 2CH teleoperation systems (solid: PEB, dashed: DFR)

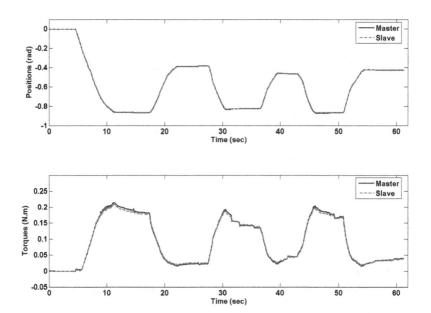

Fig. 5.11   Position and force profiles for the 3CH teleoperation system with $C_3 = 0$ and $C_5 = -1$.

and (5.12). However, as can be seen from Figures 5.8 and 5.9, contact-mode position tracking is better with DFR. With regard to h_{22}, it is important to note that because of the finite stiffness of the slave and also the backlash present in the slave's gearhead, the accuracy of $h_{22} = -X_s/F_e|_{X_m=0}$ estimates is less than that of the rest of the hybrid parameters.

As was discussed earlier, in practical implementation of the 4CH architecture, we do not consider the acceleration terms in the controllers C_1 and C_4 given in (5.21) as a noise reduction measure. Moreover, we limit our experimental study to the case where $C_6 = 0$. The reason for this is that, as reported in [52], master local force feedback ($C_6 \neq 0$) is suitable for operations in which the environment is heavier, has more damping and is stiffer than the operator's arm such as in remote excavation (as opposed to soft tissue applications).

Figure 5.11 shows the master and the slave position and torque tracking profiles for the 3CH teleoperation system in which $C_2 = 1$, $C_6 = 0$, $C_3 = 0$ and $C_5 = -1$. Figures 5.12 and 5.13 show similar profiles for the same choice of C_2 and C_6 but for $C_3 = 0.5$, $C_5 = -0.5$ (4CH system no. 1) and $C_3 = 1$, $C_5 = 0$ (4CH system no. 2), respectively. As can be seen,

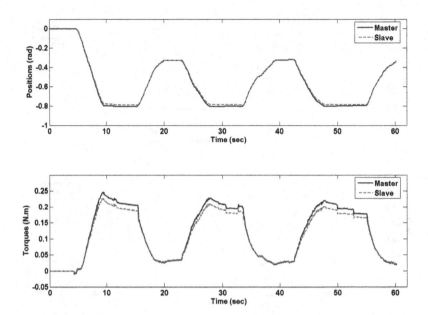

Fig. 5.12   Position and force profiles for the 4CH teleoperation system with $C_3 = 0.5$ and $C_5 = -0.5$ (4CH-1).

as the local force feedback gain at the slave is reduced (i.e., lower $|C_5|$), the contact-mode position tracking and, more significantly, force tracking performance deteriorate. This can partially be attributed to the fact that when the slave local force feedback is reduced, there is an increased level of contribution of the observed force in the slave control action $(C_3 f_h)$, which pronounces observation errors. Figures 5.11, 5.12 and 5.13 show that the 3CH architecture (with $C_3 = 0$) can lead to at least an equal level of performance compared to the 4CH architecture while it needs one less force sensor. The 3CH architecture is also superior in the sense that generally a higher gain of the slave local feedback (i.e., higher $|C_5|$) allows for a lower gain of master force feedforward (i.e., lower C_3) and consequently higher stability margin at no extra penalty on transparency. The magnitudes of the hybrid parameters of the 3CH and the two 4CH teleoperation systems are shown in Figure 5.14. As can be seen, the magnitude of h_{12} over low frequencies, which is indicative of steady-state force tracking error, increases above 0 dB as the gain of slave local force feedback is reduced. The slave local force feedback does not affect free-space position tracking as seen in h_{21} spectra of Figure 5.14.

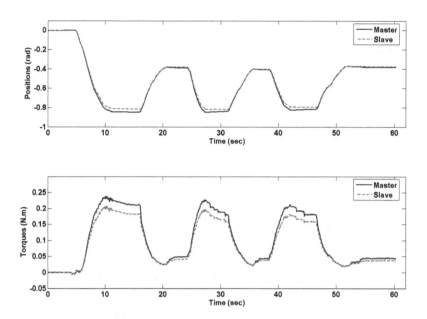

Fig. 5.13 Position and force profiles for the 4CH teleoperation system with $C_3 = 1$ and $C_5 = 0$ (4CH-2).

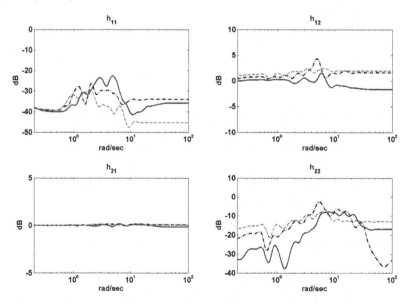

Fig. 5.14 Magnitudes of the hybrid parameters for 4CH teleoperation systems (solid: 3CH, dash-dot: 4CH-1, dashed: 4CH-2).

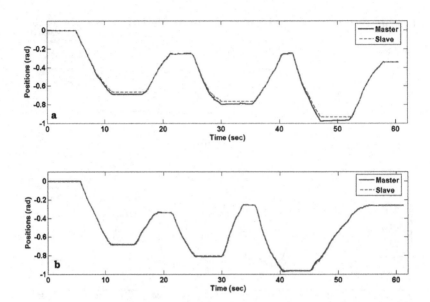

Fig. 5.15 Position profiles for (a) DFR and (b) 3CH teleoperation systems under hard contact.

Although, based on Figures 5.9 and 5.11, it seems that the DFR architecture can offer performance comparable to the 3CH architecture, it must be noted that the above experiments have been performed using a soft object made of a silicon-based tissue phantom from Chamberlain Group (http://www.thecgroup.com) placed on top of a layer of foam. Under hard contact (using a piece of wood instead of the tissue phantom), however, the DFR scheme shows degraded performance especially in terms of position tracking (Figure 5.15a) while the 3CH continues to perform satisfactorily in terms of both position tracking (Figure 5.15b) and force tracking (not shown). Due to its optimum performance and relative simplicity of implementation, the 3CH architecture is used for haptic teleoperation experiments in the next chapter.

5.4 Concluding Remarks

This chapter studied the stability and transparency of 2-channel and 4-channel bilateral teleoperation control architectures from both stability and transparency points of view. Using a haptics-capable master-slave test-bed, it was found that slave/environment force measurements can significantly improve teleoperation transparency in a 2-channel architecture. In contrast to 2-channel architectures, a sufficient number of design parameters in the 4-channel architecture enables it to achieve ideal transparency. However, as a result of the stability-performance tradeoff, the stability of the ideally transparent 4-channel system critically depends on exact implementation of the control laws and having exact model of the teleoperation system. On the other hand, local force feedback terms in the 4-channel architecture can be used to increase the stability and performance robustness of the teleoperation system against non-idealities in bilateral control implementation. The theoretical results were validated by experiments conducted using our haptics-capable master-slave setup developed for an endoscopic surgery environment.

Chapter 6

Substitution for Haptic Feedback

6.1 Introduction

For haptic feedback of instrument/tissue interactions to the surgeon's hand during master-slave operation, the minimum requirement is to have a force-reflective human-machine interface (HMI). Moreover, it is desirable to have a force sensor on the slave robot for measuring the instrument/tissue interaction, which can lead to more reliable haptic feedback than position error based force reflection. In minimally invasive surgery, such a force sensor needs to be mounted on the section of the surgical instrument that goes past the port and inside the patient in order to avoid corrupting the readings with friction and other disturbances at the entry port. This requirement complicates the design of the robotic arm, creates sterilization issues, and raises the cost of the system. Consequently, the addition of a force sensor on the slave surgical robot has so far been avoided in today's surgical systems (e.g., the da Vinci system from Intuitive Surgical Inc., Sunnyvale, CA). The result is that in the current surgical systems, due to limitations in the present actuator and sensor technology, there are only flows of surgeon's hand motions and camera vision data from the master side to the slave side and vice versa and there is no haptic feedback. However, the absence of haptic feedback to the surgeon in robot-assisted surgery is a safety concern and a cause of errors [117]. For instance, in a study involving minimally invasive cholecystectomy, it was observed that inappropriate and excessive application of force was one of the main causes of perforation of the gallbladder [68]. Such a safety concern is especially significant if visual feedback to the surgeon is degraded, e.g., if fluids from the patient's body cloud the camera lens or the instruments leave the limited field of view of the endoscopic camera.

At the other end of the spectrum, a question that arises is, if a haptic HMI is not available, can slave-side force measurement be of any help with regard to improving surgical outcomes? It seems that at least in the short term and for some applications involving robotic surgery, it may be useful and even more cost-effective to provide substitute modes of sensory feedback to the surgeon, e.g., by graphical representation of haptic information. While force feedback remains a more intuitive means of relaying haptic information to the user, substitution for haptic feedback may be able to provide sufficient feedback of an instrument's contact with tissue under certain conditions. To verify this, in Section 6.2 we examine the potential of graphical feedback of instrument/tissue interaction to the surgeon. Using our master-slave testbed (Section 5.3.1), experiments involving a lump localization task are conducted and the performance of human subjects is compared for different modalities of instrument/tissue contact feedback.

The second question that is addressed in this chapter is the following: The currently available surgical systems provide visual feedback but no haptic feedback to the surgeon, yet surgeons have relied on visual feedback for performing complicated interventions such as coronary artery bypass grafting [126]. Can haptic feedback or sensory substitution for haptic feedback offer any help specially if visual feedback is of a poor quality? For this question, in Section 6.3, user performance is compared for a telemanipulated soft tissue stiffness discrimination task when users are provided with visual feedback, haptic feedback, and graphical substitution for haptic feedback.

First, the benefits and requirements of sensory substitution for haptic feedback are reviewed.

Requirements Haptic feedback can be substituted in more than one way, for instance by providing the surgeon with auditory, graphical, or vibro-tactile cues about instrument/tissue contacts. The substitute feedback channel is required to be intuitive and provide a straightforward mapping to haptic information. It should have minimum background noise, and have a fairly large bandwidth (communication capacity). In the context of surgical applications, substitution of haptic information by auditory signals (in the form of different auditory tones) is not favored by surgeons as it can interfere with the conversations within the surgical team and provides only single-event reports rather than continuous real-time information about instrument/tissue contacts. Surgeons are not in general familiar with vibro-tactile inputs (in the form of different vibration intensities) ei-

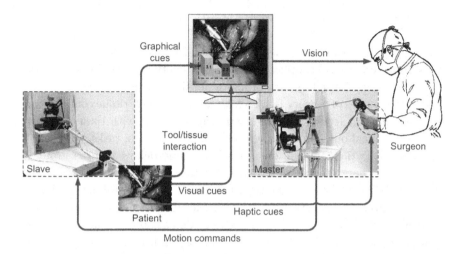

Fig. 6.1   Visual substitution/augmentation for haptic feedback.

ther. However, graphical display of haptic information, "graphical force feedback", as overlaid on or beside the endoscope view can relay haptic information to the surgeon simply based on the size and/or color of the visual stimuli. Figure 6.1 shows how haptic feedback can be substituted or augmented by the corresponding visual information in a master-slave surgical procedure.

Benefits   Study of the effect of substitution for haptic feedback for a peg-in-hole insertion task has shown that both visual feedback and vibro-tactile feedback of haptic information can reduce the peak forces compared to the case where no feedback of haptic information is provided to the users [29]. Moreover, visual substitution for haptic feedback has been found to improve a user's sensitivity for detecting small forces by allowing the use of high feedback gains without slowing down hand movements [89]. These studies have not been performed in the context of surgical applications. For manual operation and robotic teleoperation of a surgical knot tying task, the forces applied in the robotic mode were closer to the forces applied in the manual mode when the users were provided with auditory/graphical substitution of haptic information [74]. It would be interesting to see the difference between haptic feedback and graphical substitution for haptic feedback in the robotic mode itself.

6.2   Graphical Substitution for Haptic Feedback

As discussed in Section 6.1, the lack of haptic feedback in the current surgical systems can cause complications and is a safety concern. As a solution
to the problems caused by lack of haptic feedback, it is hypothesized that
alternative modes of sensory feedback about instrument/tissue contacts can
provide sufficient feedback of an instrument's contact with tissue and can
improve surgical outcomes during robot-assisted surgical tasks.

In teleoperation applications with large time delays such as ground-
to-space teleoperation where it is difficult to compensate for the adverse
effect of the large delay on haptic teleoperation system stability and performance, graphical substitution for haptic feedback is a viable alternative.
Moreover, if the user interface has force reflection capability in fewer degrees
of freedom than those of the task, partial force reflection may destabilize
the teleoperation system [145], in which case replacing haptic feedback by
graphical feedback is useful. In the following, haptic feedback and graphical
haptic feedback are compared in terms of their capability in transmitting
critical task-related information to the user.

6.2.1   *Case study: Lump localization task*

6.2.1.1   *Experiment design*

Six subjects (2 males and 4 females) aged 24-34 participated in our experiments. The subjects were engineering students with little to average
exposure to haptic feedback and graphical substitution for haptic feedback.
The task was to locate a rigid lump, which was embedded in an unknown
location in a finite-stiffness homogeneous tissue model made from rubber.
Lump localization was based on exploring the model and receiving haptic or
graphical feedback using the master-slave setup described in Section 5.3.1
(see Figure 6.2). The graphical cues about the levels of tool/tissue interaction forces were generated by an array of light-emitting diodes forming
a bar indicator for the magnitudes of forces. The lump was placed in one
of five locations at approximately 34, 65, 92, 124 and 158 degrees with respect to the horizon. The size of the lump (5 mm) was chosen such that
users could detect the lump in a reasonable amount of time. Each lump
localization trial started from orienting the master handle (and the slave's
end-effector) such that it was horizontal followed by twisting the handle to
explore the tissue until the handle was again horizontal on the other side

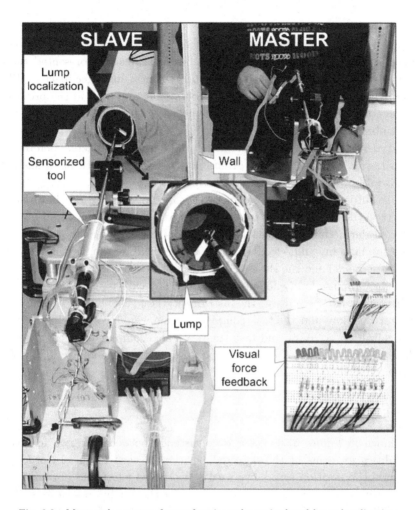

Fig. 6.2 Master-slave setup for performing telemanipulated lump localization.

(equal to a wrist rotation of +180° for the user).

The subjects' primary goal was defined as pinpointing the lump by centering the slave end-effector on it. The subjects were told that the task completion time was a secondary performance metric that needed to be minimized, yet they could take their time if it helped to minimize the primary performance metric (i.e., localization error). This is different from most of the previous studies on sensory substitution, which have considered task completion time as the only metric for performance comparisons. A task was considered complete upon the subject's verbal signal that the lump was found.

Each subject performed two sets of tests with a short break between them. In each test, each of the five lump locations was presented twice to the subject: once in the presence of graphical force feedback (GFF) about the levels of instrument/tissue interaction, and once in the presence of force feedback (FF). Therefore, in each test there were 10 trials (i.e., 10 combinations of lump location and feedback mode). The trials within a test were presented in a randomized order to the subjects. Before the experiments, each subject was given 3-4 practice trials until he or she felt comfortable with the operation of the master-slave system.

The subjects did not have camera vision from the slave side in order to keep tissue deformation cues from playing a role in lump localization – we do not consider nodules that can be visually detected through moving tissue. Also, to mask any audio feedback that can result from the friction between the tissue model and the slave's end-effector, the subjects wore headphones that played music loud enough to mask out any external sounds.

In each trial of each test, the instrument/tissue contact forces, the end-effector position, and the task completion time were recorded. In addition to localization accuracy and task times, we also compared the energy supplied to tissue as lower energy corresponds to less trauma and probably less tissue damage.

6.2.1.2   *Results*

As shown in Figure 6.3a, there is consistency between the two feedback modalities in terms of the detected position of each lump. In order to compare the position errors, we used a two-tailed t-test and obtained the probability of the null hypothesis $\mu_1 = \mu_2$ for the five lump locations. The probability of the results assuming the null hypothesis for lump locations 1 to 5 were $p = 0.00019$, $p = 0.028$, $p = 0.515$, $p = 0.413$, and $p = 0.714$, respectively. These results indicate that for lump locations 3, 4, and 5, there is no significant difference in mean localization error between GFF and FF. This might be partly due to the fact that the subjects experienced some difficulty in localizing the first two lump positions as they were too close to the starting point of the slave. In order to further investigate the accuracy of lump localization, we performed a one-way ANOVA test (Appendix D.2) on the localization error statistics of the five lump locations for both GFF and FF ($F(4, 82) = 0.4589$, $p = 0.766$ for GFF; and $F(4, 82) = 3.31$, $p = 0.014$ for FF). These results indicate that the localization error means

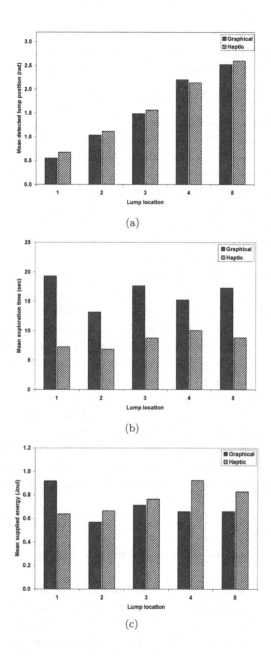

Fig. 6.3 (a) Mean detected lump position (rad); (b) mean exploration time (sec); (c) mean energy supplied to the tissue (Joule).

do not vary significantly across the five lump locations for GFF, but do vary significantly for FF.

Figure 6.3b depicts the statistics of the time (seconds) taken to localize a lump in each of the five locations. As a general observation, the mean localization time is significantly longer with GFF than with FF (267%, 192%, 201%, 151%, and 195% longer for lump locations 1 to 5, respectively). Right-tailed t-tests between GFF and FF for localization times of each lump location confirm this observation ($p = 4.515 \times 10^{-5}$, $p = 0.0013$, $p = 0.00017$, $p = 0.00036$, and $p = 0.00011$ for lump locations 1 to 5, respectively). In order to investigate the effect of lump positions on the exploration time, a one-way ANOVA test was conducted on the exploration time statistics of the five lump locations for both GFF and FF ($F(4, 82) = 1.119$, $p = 0.353$ for GFF; and $F(4, 82) = 2.579$, $p = 0.043$ for FF). These results confirm the fact that the exploration time means do not vary significantly across the five lump locations for GFF but vary significantly for FF.

Figure 6.3c depicts the statistics of the energy (Joules; calculated as $\int_0^T f(t)v(t)\mathrm{d}t$ where T, f, and v are the task completion time, the contact force, and the slave's velocity, respectively) supplied to the tissue during lump localization for each of the five lump locations with GFF and with FF. Excluding the first location, FF-based lump localization seems to supply more energy to tissue in comparison to GFF. Again, we tested this hypothesis by means of a right-tailed t-test ($p = 0.006$, $p = 0.141$, $p = 0.204$, $p = 0.001$, and $p = 0.003$ for lump locations 1 to 5, respectively). These results show that the mean of the energy supplied to tissue under GFF and FF varies significantly for lump locations 1, 4 and 5. A one-way ANOVA test for the energy over the five lump locations yielded $F(4, 82) = 2.96$, $p = 0.0244$ for GFF and $F(4, 82) = 2.812$, $p = 0.0306$ for FF, which indicate significant variations across the five lump locations for both modalities.

6.2.1.3 *Discussion*

The following trends were observed in lump localization performance with GFF and FF:

The subjects were 100% successful in localizing the lumps under both GFF and FF with position errors significantly less than half the average distance between the lumps. No consistent trend was observed in favor of either approach with respect to the localization accuracy except for a weak tendency for better accuracy with GFF. Considering the lower system complexity required for implementing GFF, even an equivalent level of accuracy can be regarded as an advantage for GFF. However, it must be noted that with GFF, a user can perform well only if the sensitivity and resolution of the graphical display is sufficiently high so that small variations in the reflected force become discernible.

The exploration time for GFF is considerably longer than for FF. This observation is justifiable given the fact that with GFF, the subjects have to constantly refer to the graphical display in order to detect a significant variation in the contact force profile, which corresponds to a lump. Therefore, while providing graphical feedback about instrument/tissue interaction is useful for the purpose of lump localization, the corresponding task times are longer due to the need for cognitive processing by the users. This conclusion is consistent with previous results for teleoperation of non-surgical tasks [89]. From the user's point of view, GFF's moderate need for human processing and interpretation may be a major drawback particularly for lengthy procedures or for dexterous tasks, in which the user has to keep track of several graphical indicators and switch his/her attention between them without getting distracted from the main surgical task (sensory overload).

With regard to the energy supplied to the tissue by the users, the results are not consistently in favor of either GFF or FF. The higher levels of supplied energy under FF for two locations (out of five) seem to be a result of the fact that the localization ability under FF is proportional to the slave's velocity. In contrast, the slower the slave moves, the higher the localization ability will be under GFF.

6.3 Multi-Modal Contact Cues

Internet-based signal transmission and video streaming is increasingly becoming the technology of choice for a wide range of applications including unilateral and bilateral teleoperation [148, 112]. In this method of transmission, the video quality can be easily affected by network congestion resulting in poor video quality at the human operator side [151].

Degraded visual conditions caused by IP network impairments or other factors such as signal-to-noise degradation in wireless communication or depth perception difficulties in 2-D vision can make it difficult to prevent tissue damage in the absence of haptic sensation for the surgeon. In this section, we study the effects of visual, haptic and graphical cues about tool/tissue interactions on user's performance for a typical surgical task.

While the inclusion of haptic feedback in a virtual-reality surgical simulator for a tissue holding task has been shown to help the user when visual feedback is impeded [91], our goal is to study how effectively the graphical or haptic cues can replace corrupted visual feedback in master-slave surgical teleoperation.

6.3.1 *Case study: Tissue stiffness discrimination Task*

6.3.1.1 *Experiment Design*

Using the master-slave system, teleoperation experiments were conducted in which the task is to discriminate between any two soft tissues with different stiffnesses through tele-robotic palpation. The motivation for studying this task is given by the fact that tissue palpation is one of the ways to detect cancerous tissue, which has a different stiffness compared to healthy tissue. Several contact feedback modalities are compared in terms of their capability in transmitting critical task-related information to the user.

In our experimental scenario, the visual link consisted of a 320 × 240 webcam-provided image, which is transmitted from the slave side to the master side via a H.323-based NetMeeting Internet video-conferencing application at a rate of 14 frames per second. The communication media was a 1000T-base Ethernet network.

Six subjects (3 males and 3 females) aged 24-34 participated in our experiments. The subjects had little to average exposure to haptic and graphical cues and average experience with the master-slave system. The subjects' primary goal was defined as distinguishing between different tissues in terms of their relative stiffness. After a tissue sample was presented to the subject and probed, it was replaced with a different or the same tissue sample upon the subject's verbal signal. The subjects would also verbally signify the completion of the task.

The subjects received visual, haptic, graphical, or graphical plus haptic cues about the level of tool/tissue interactions forces as the tool indented the soft tissue (see Figure 6.4). Since our intention was to study the utility of haptic and graphical feedback under degraded or suppressed visual conditions, camera vision from the slave side was switched off when the subjects received haptic and/or graphical cues so that visual cues did not play a role.

In each trial, one out of the above-mentioned four different feedback modalities and a combination of two out of three different tissue samples

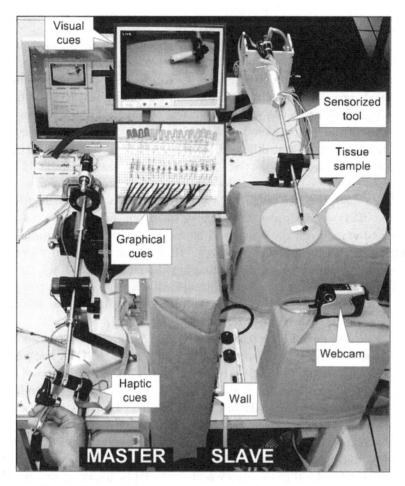

Fig. 6.4 Master-slave setup for performing telemanipulated tissue stiffness discrimination task.

(two different tissues or the same tissue twice) were presented to the subject. In total, each subject made 16 trials (i.e., 16 combinations of feedback modality and tissue pair randomly selected out of the 24 possible combinations). The trials were presented in a randomized order to the subjects. Before the experiments, each subject was given 3-4 practice trials until he or she felt comfortable with the operation of the master-slave system. Each palpation trial started from orienting the master handle (the slave's end-effector) in vertical (horizontal) position followed by twisting the handle to explore the tissue (user's wrist rotation angle $\in [0\ 90°]$).

6.3.1.2   *Results*

The test results for the palpation task are shown in Figure 6.5 in the form of bar graphs of mean values. Figure 6.5a shows the trials' success rate for the four different feedback modes. As can be seen, graphical cueing is the most successful modality for tissue stiffness discrimination. To further investigate this, first a one-way ANOVA test was applied to the success rate statistics of the feedback modes ($F(3, 92) = 1.426$, $p = 0.2401$), which did not indicate a significant difference among the success rate statistics. Due to the pass/fail nature of the tests (1: successful; 0: unsuccessful) and for a more elaborate analysis, we used separate t-tests between different pairs of feedback modes. A two-tailed t-test between graphical and visual feedback modes ($t(24) = 1.163$, $p = 0.257$) shows no significant difference. A two-tailed t-test between the visual and haptic modes indicates no significant difference ($t(24) = 2.069$, $p = 0.538$). However, a right-tailed t-test between the graphical and haptic feedback modes ($t(24) = 1.813$, $p = 0.0415$) indicates higher success rate for graphical feedback compared to haptic feedback. Another two-tailed t-test between haptic and haptic plus graphical feedback modes showed them to be almost identical ($p > 0.5$).

The bar graph of Figure 6.5b represents the mean values of task completion times (seconds) for different feedback modes. An ANOVA test for the four feedback modes ($F(3, 92) = 0.7627$, $p = 0.5178$) shows that there is no significant difference among the average task times. However, a two-tailed t-test ($t(24) = 2.069$, $p = 0.0285$) shows that the task completion times are longer under visual feedback than haptic feedback.

Figure 6.5c shows the mean values of the energy supplied to tissue (Joules) under the four feedback modes. This graph indicates that the haptic plus graphical mode (very closely followed by haptic mode) and the visual mode supplied the lowest and the highest energy to tissues, respectively. An ANOVA test confirms significant difference between the haptic, graphical and visual modes from the energy point of view ($F(2, 69) = 6.3806$ corresponding to $p = 0.000241$, which based on 5% level of ruling for p-values implies significantly different mean energies). In order to further study the closeness of the mean supplied energy under the visual and graphical feedback modes, a right-tailed t-test ($t(24) = 2.247$ corresponding to $p = 0.01725$) shows that visual cues supply significantly higher energy to tissue. A two-tailed t-test ($t(24) = 2.069$, $p = 0.0037$) confirms that the mean supplied energy for the visual mode is significantly higher than that for the haptic mode. A right-tailed t-test between the graphical and haptic

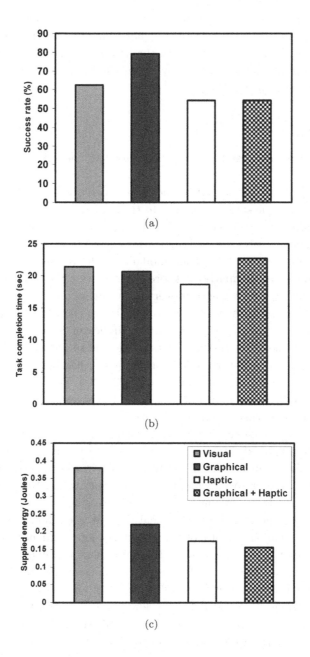

Fig. 6.5   (a) Mean success rate; (b) mean completion time (sec); (c) mean energy supplied to the tissue (Joule).

modes ($t(24) = 2.069$, $p = 0.025$) shows that the mean supplied energy for the graphical mode is significantly higher than that for the haptic mode. Finally, a right-tailed t-test between the haptic and the haptic plus graphical modes confirms that the null hypothesis $\mu_1 = \mu_2$ holds ($t(24) = 0.7355$ corresponding to $p = 0.2347$).

6.3.1.3   *Discussion*

After analyzing the results of the palpation trials, the following trends were observed:

Since a subject had to decide whether the two tissue samples were "similar", "the first one softer compared to the second one", and "the first one harder compared to the second one", the chance level was 33%. Therefore, all of the success rates are well above this chance level. As for the relative success rate of different feedback modalities, the results show that for a task involving the comparison of force/deformation tissue characteristics, graphical cueing is advantageous over haptic cueing. One reason for the superior performance achieved with graphical cues compared to haptic cues is that the sensitivity of a graphical force indicator is only limited by the resolution of the force measurements, while the sensitivity of haptic rendering is limited in nature (0.5 N or 7% is the just-noticeable difference for force sensing by the human hand) [122, 18]. The superiority of the graphical mode comes along with the benefit of simplicity of its implementation. On the downside, one should bear in mind that the domain of tasks that can benefit from graphical cues is not very extensive as with increased task complexity/dexterity (e.g., increase in a task's number of degrees of freedom), there can be a tremendous increase in the cognitive processing required by the user. An advantage of haptic cues is that they are intuitive and require the least amount of cognitive processing.

As for the success rate with visual cues, it was observed during the experiments that the depth of tissue indentation could not be precisely quantified by the subjects. While this may make one expect the success rate to be significantly lower for visual cueing compared to the graphical cueing, this was not corroborated by the two-tailed t-test – a fact that may be attributed to the relatively low number of trials (a total of 96 trials as a result of having 6 subjects and 16 trials per subject; an average of 24 trials per feedback modality). The success rate for visual cues strongly depends on the video's information content, which in turn can be attributed to various task-dependent and task-independent factors ranging from network conditions for IP-based video streaming to the camera's angle of view. For example, task performance might be seriously degraded if critical movements of the task are orthogonal to the camera view causing depth perception problems. The close success rates for the visual and haptic modes show that haptic feedback can effectively replace a degraded visual cue.

Although one might have expected the graphical plus haptic mode to result in a significantly higher success rate compared to haptic feedback, this was not corroborated by the two-tailed t-test that was done. In practice, it was observed that during the subjects' simultaneous exposure to the haptic and graphical cues in this particular task, they had strong tendencies toward the haptic portion, which made the statistics quite similar to those of the pure haptic mode.

With respect to task completion time, haptic feedback performs better than visual feedback. Although one's expectation would be that haptic cues result in much shorter task times, in practice this was not the case due to the fact that the tissue stiffnesses were not significantly different and subjects needed to palpate each tissue usually more than once.

The worst performance in terms of supplying energy and consequently incurring damage/injury to tissue was provided by the visual cueing mode. The reason is that a subject had to supply a significant amount of energy before tissue deformations were quantifiable. As a result, the distance between the visual mode and the other modalities with respect to the supplied energy to tissue is quite noticeable. Therefore, the haptic mode can also effectively replace a corrupted visual cue from an energy point of view.

6.4 Concluding Remarks

Using our haptics-capable master-slave testbed, for localization of a lump embedded in soft tissue, performance comparisons were made for situations in which haptic feedback is substituted by graphical display of haptic information. It was observed that the localization accuracy is comparable for both feedback modalities, meaning that in cases where a haptic user interface is not available, graphical force feedback can adequately and cost-effectively substitute for haptic feedback. However, this comes at the expense of longer task completion times for graphical feedback. Moreover, we compared users' performance under visual, haptic, graphical, and graphical plus haptic feedback modalities for a soft-tissue palpation task. The goal was to study how effectively the graphical or haptic cues can replace a corrupted visual cue. It was found that graphical cueing and haptic cueing led to respectively a higher and an equal rate of success in discriminating between two tissue samples with different stiffnesses compared to the visual mode, while the visual mode incurs the highest risk of tissue damage due to excessive tissue deformation.

Chapter 7

Bilateral Teleoperation Control Under Time Delay

7.1 Introduction

As discussed in the previous chapters, master-slave teleoperation is greatly enhanced if some form of kinesthetic feedback about the interaction occurring between the slave robot and the remote environment is provided to the human operator through the master robot. Such systems are called "bilateral" because information flows in two directions between the operator and the remote environment. However, communication latencies exist if there is a large distance between the local and the remote sites. Such delayed kinesthetic feedback can pose serious problems to a bilateral teleoperation system [120, 49, 64]. A comprehensive survey of the literature on time delay compensation methods can be found in [5, 57].

The passivity-based approach has been shown to be an efficient method for stabilizing a two-channel (2CH) teleoperation architecture (involving transmission of only one quantity from the master to the slave and vice versa) independent of transmission delays at the expense of degraded transparency [3]. A reformulation of this idea led to the introduction of the wave transformation approach [101, 102] , which provides a flexible design and analysis tool for 2CH teleoperation systems. In this chapter, first we will utilize the wave transformation technique in a 2CH teleoperation architecture which is based upon kinesthetic feedback of direct force measurements at the slave side. To this end, the following steps are taken:

- In order to carry out an in-depth study of stability and transparency of a teleoperation system in the presence of time delay, the passivity-based approach proposed in [3] is extended and admittance-type and hybrid-type two-port network models (architectures) based on different choices of wave transformation arrangements are introduced, which warrant different teleoperation control configurations. In both cases (admittance-type and hybrid-type), the teleoperation system configuration is affected by the presence or absence of force sensing in the system.

- Stability of admittance-type configurations is examined using a passivity framework analysis of an end-to-end model of the teleoperation system (the master+communication channel+the slave). It is shown that stability can be maintained in the presence of force sensing, and closed-form conditions for absolutely stable operation of different configurations are derived. To the best of our knowledge, this issue has not been addressed previously.

- Our results show that for haptic teleoperation applications, practical considerations suggest that it is more advantageous to use a hybrid-type architecture instead of an admittance-type architecture. Moreover, experimental results indicate that slave-side force measurements considerably improve transparency compared to the position error-based approach in the hybrid-type architecture.

On the other hand, it has been demonstrated that the extra "degrees of freedom" (control parameters) in the four-channel (4CH) architecture make it the best teleoperation system from a transparency point of view when there are no time delays [79, 153]. The missing component is stabilization of the 4CH architecture under time delay without imposing any additional penalty on the system transparency. The following main issues are discussed in this chapter with respect to delay compensation in the 4CH architecture:

- A new 4CH architecture has been proposed in this chapter which uses wave transformation for making the delayed communication channel passive. In order to incorporate the wave theory in the 4CH bilateral control architecture, appropriate linear combinations of forces and velocities at the input and output of the passivated delayed communication channel are introduced such that the corresponding pseudo-power signals comply with passivity formalism.

- The proposed architecture is flexible enough to achieve ideal transparency in the presence of time delay. We have derived the conditions for realizing this property. Moreover, a stability study for the ideally transparent system is conducted and the corresponding stability condition is derived.

- We have proposed wave-based 3-channel (3CH) architectures, which are derived from the 4CH architecture through appropriate selection control gains. The cited bilateral teleoperation control architectures are capable of offering satisfactory sub-optimum transparency with significantly less implementation complexity.

The theoretical work presented in this chapter is also supported by experimental results.

7.2 Passivity and Absolute Stability

We assume the following single DOF equations of motions for the master and the slave manipulators throughout our work:

$$M_m \ddot{x}_m = -f_m + f_h \qquad M_s \ddot{x}_s = f_s - f_e \qquad (7.1)$$

where M_m and M_s are the master and slave inertias, f_m and f_s are the master and slave control actions, and x_m and x_s are the master and slave positions. Also, f_h and f_e represent the interaction forces between the operator's hand and the master, and the slave and the remote environment, respectively. As it was discussed in Section 5.2, by considering velocities and forces in a teleoperation system as currents and voltages, an equivalent electrical circuit representation of the system can be obtained. This equivalent circuit representation can be expressed by the following hybrid model:

$$\begin{bmatrix} F_h \\ -\dot{X}_s \end{bmatrix} = \begin{bmatrix} h_{11} & h_{12} \\ h_{21} & h_{22} \end{bmatrix} \cdot \begin{bmatrix} \dot{X}_m \\ F_e \end{bmatrix}$$

To achieve ideally transparent bilateral teleoperation system in the presence of time delay, the concept of transparency in [79, 52] can be further extended to the delayed kinematic correspondence and the delayed interaction force correspondence ($\dot{X}_s = e^{-sT}\dot{X}_m$ and $F_h = e^{-sT}F_e$, respectively). Consequently, the hybrid matrix of a delayed ideally transparent teleoperation system takes the following form:

$$H = \begin{bmatrix} 0 & e^{-sT} \\ -e^{-sT} & 0 \end{bmatrix} \qquad (7.2)$$

7.2.1 *Passivity-based time delay compensation*

In the presence of a time delay, the ideally transparent bilateral teleoperation system outlined by (7.2) has the following scattering matrix:

$$S = \begin{bmatrix} -\tanh(sT) & \mathrm{sech}(sT) \\ \mathrm{sech}(sT) & \tanh(sT) \end{bmatrix} \tag{7.3}$$

It can be shown that $\bar{\sigma}(S)$ for this scattering matrix is unbounded, consequently (according to Theorem 5.4) this system cannot maintain stability. In practice, stability and transparency are competing issues in a teleoperation system [79]. Therefore, one can intuitively argue that $\bar{\sigma}(S) = 1$ is the optimum choice for maintaining stability while the system operates with the best achievable transparency possible. A physical interpretation for a two-port network with $\bar{\sigma}(S) = 1$ is the ideal transmission line with time delay, which can be represented by the following pair of hybrid and scattering matrices:

$$H = \begin{bmatrix} \tanh(sT) & \mathrm{sech}(sT) \\ -\mathrm{sech}(sT) & \tanh(sT) \end{bmatrix} \quad S = \begin{bmatrix} 0 & e^{-sT} \\ e^{-sT} & 0 \end{bmatrix} \tag{7.4}$$

Comparing scattering matrices in equations (7.3) and (7.4), it can be seen that in the delayed transmission line, stability has been attained at the expense of degraded transparency. Based on this argument, the following control law was proposed in [3], which passivates a communication channel with time delay in a two-channel bilateral teleoperation system:

$$F_{md} = F_s e^{-sT} + n^2 (\dot{X}_m - \dot{X}_{sd} e^{-sT})$$
$$\dot{X}_{sd} = \dot{X}_m e^{-sT} + n^{-2} (F_{md} e^{-sT} - F_s) \tag{7.5}$$

An energy-based approach, which yields the same results in a more physically-motivated manner, was proposed in [101]. A pair of wave variables (u, v) is defined, based on a pair of standard power variables $(\dot{x}, f)$, by the following (Figure 7.1):

$$u = \frac{b\dot{x} + f}{\sqrt{2b}} \quad v = \frac{b\dot{x} - f}{\sqrt{2b}} \tag{7.6}$$

where u denotes the right moving wave while v denotes the left moving wave. The characteristic wave impedance b is a positive constant and assumes the role of a tuning parameter.

Depending on the choice of input/output pairs from the four variables in equations (7.6), we distinguish four two-port network models (i.e., architectures) for the delay-compensated communication channel. These four architectures correspond to well-known representations of a two-port network as an impedance matrix, an admittance matrix, a hybrid matrix, or an inverse hybrid matrix. Among these four architectures, in order to have

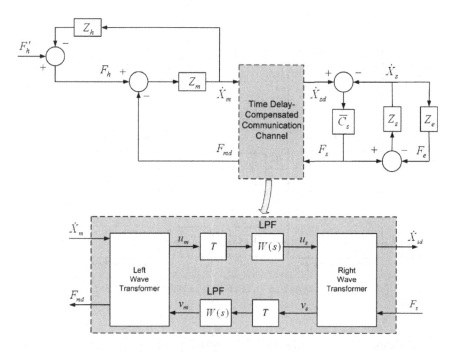

Fig. 7.1 Wave-based delay compensated 2CH position error based teleoperator.

a stiff slave, we are interested in the two cases in which the slave is under position control, namely namely the admittance-type (Figure 7.2a) and the hybrid-type (Figure 7.2b) delay-compensated channels. In both architectures, the time delay T has been assumed to be constant and equal in both directions. In the admittance-type delay-compensated channel, the master and the slave velocities have been taken as outputs of the overall two-port network. In the hybrid-type, however, the slave velocity and the force transmitted to the master side are outputs. In each architecture, based on the absence or presence of force sensing at the master and/or the slave sides, two control configurations are possible; namely position error-based (PEB) or kinesthetic force-based (KFB).

In practice, a wave-based teleoperation system performance can be degraded due to a number of reasons, among which are discrete implementation of continuous-time control laws and significant variations in the operator's behavior or the environment impedance. The performance is particularly degraded for large time delays where high frequency oscillations appear in the teleoperation system. The idea of filtering the wave variables

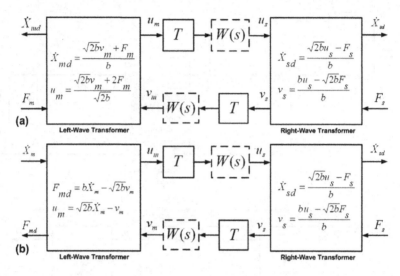

Fig. 7.2   (a) Admittance-type and (b) hybrid-type delay-compensated communication channels.

(wave-domain lowpass filtering) was initially suggested in [101] for noise reduction and frequency shaping, especially when the proposed impedance matching scheme fails to achieve the goal of transparency improvement. In continuation of this work, [133] compared the performance of impedance matching and wave filtering. In this research, we use lowpass filters $W(s)$ in the wave domain according to Figure 7.2 and obtain the corresponding stability conditions.

7.3   2-Channel Architectures

7.3.1   *Admittance-type configurations*

7.3.1.1   *APEB and filtered APEB*

A wave-based Admittance-type Position-Error Based (APEB) teleoperation system is illustrated in Figure 7.3a. In this system, let us take $M_m = M_s = M$ and PD position controllers $C_m(s) = C_s(s) = (k_d s + k_p)/s$ used at the master and the slave. The resulting teleoperation system has a scattering matrix that is both reciprocal and symmetric. As a result, investigating system stability using Theorem 5.4 is analytically tractable.

In the neighbourhood of $T = 0$ (fairly small time delays), by using a first

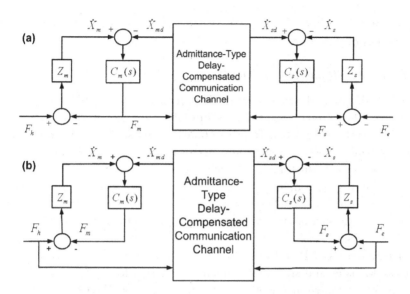

Fig. 7.3   Wave-based admittance-type teleoperation systems: (a) APEB; (b) AKFB.

order Padé approximation for the exponential terms in the characteristic polynomial of the S matrix, it can be inferred that the sufficient condition for S to be RHP analytic is $k_d > 0$ and $k_p > 0$. The singular values of the scattering matrix for the APEB teleoperation system are:

$$\sigma_1, \sigma_2 = \left| \frac{(A_1 - B_1 + C_1 - D_1)e^{-sT} \pm (A_1 + B_1 - C_1 - D_1)}{(A_1 - B_1 - C_1 + D_1)e^{-sT} \pm (A_1 + B_1 + C_1 + D_1)} \right| \quad (7.7)$$

where $A_1 = Mbs^2 + bk_ds + bk_p$, $B_1 = Ms(k_ds + k_p)$, $C_1 = k_ds + k_p$ and $D_1 = bs$. Therefore, condition (b) for stability leads to:

$$2b^2 k_d \omega^2 [1 \pm \cos(\omega T)] \geq 0 \quad (7.8)$$

Since $k_d > 0$, both of the inequalities in (7.8) hold regardless of ω or T. If wave-domain low pass filters are utilized in the APEB teleoperation system, the stability conditions will be (a) $k_d > 0$ and $k_p > 0$ as sufficient conditions, and (b) the singular values of the new scattering matrix will be the same as (7.7) if e^{-sT} is replaced by $e^{-sT}W(s)$, giving the following stability condition:

$$\frac{L^2[k_d \omega^2 (b + k_d) + k_p^2] + 2bk_d}{2bk_d \sqrt{1 + L^2}} \geq |\cos(\omega T + \varphi)| \quad (7.9)$$

where $\tan(\varphi) = L$, $W(s) = (Ls + 1)^{-1}$, $L = (2\pi f_{cut})^{-1}$, and f_{cut} is the cut-off frequency of the first-order lowpass filters. The above condition defines a region of stability for a filtered APEB teleoperation system. For $L = 0$, (7.9) simplifies to (7.8).

7.3.1.2 *AKFB and filtered AKFB*

Both Anderson and Spong [3] and Niemeyer and Slotine [101] have avoided the use of force sensor measurements in bilateral teleoperation control due to the questions which may arise about the passivity of the whole system. In this chapter, a new two-channel wave-based teleoperation architecture is proposed which uses force sensing at both the master and the slave ends. In this section, we show that incorporating force sensor measurements in a time-delay teleoperation control algorithm does not necessarily destablize the system and we derive corresponding absolute stability conditions. Figure 7.3b depicts a wave-based Admittance-type Kinesthetic Force Based (AKFB) teleoperation configuration, in which measurements of hand-master and slave-environment interaction forces are used. Due to reciprocity and symmetry of its scattering matrix, an AKFB teleoperation system can be studied analytically. Similar to the APEB configuration, a sufficient condition set for meeting first criterion of Theorem 5.4 is $k_d > 0$ and $k_p > 0$. For the second criterion,

$$\sigma_1, \sigma_2 = \left| \frac{(A_2 + B_2 - C_2)e^{-sT} \pm (A_2 - B_2 - C_2)}{(A_2 - B_2 + C_2)e^{-sT} \pm (A_2 + B_2 + C_2)} \right| \tag{7.10}$$

where $A_2 = Mbs^2 + bk_ds + bk_p$, $B_2 = k_ds + k_p$, and $C_2 = bs$. The stability condition is given by

$$\frac{b}{\sqrt{b^2 + \omega^2 M^2}} \geq |\cos(\omega T - \varphi)| \tag{7.11}$$

where $\tan(\varphi) = \omega M/b$. In this configuration, the region of stability is more limited in comparison to APEB. However, absolute stability can be achieved through proper selection of system parameters. For instance, choosing the system's parameters such that $\omega M \ll b$ sufficiently ensures criterion (7.11). If we make use of lowpass filters in AKFB, the singular values of the new scattering matrix can be obtained from (7.10) through replacing e^{-sT} by $e^{-sT}W(s)$. In this way, the corresponding stability condition set is:

$$\frac{\omega^2 L^2(bk_d - Mk_p + k_d^2) + L^2k_p^2 + 2bk_d}{2k_d\sqrt{(1 + \omega^2 L^2)(b^2 + \omega^2 M^2)}} \geq |\cos(\omega T - \varphi)| \tag{7.12}$$

where $\tan(\varphi) = \omega(M - bL)/(M\omega^2 L + b)$. Similar to (7.11), (7.12) can be also satisfied through proper choice of the relevant parameters.

7.3.1.3 *Implementation issues*

Our interest in hybrid-type teleoperation configurations stems from a tuning disadvantage of the admittance-type configurations. From the controller tuning point of view, assuming an APEB teleoperation system without time delay, the closed-loop control law at the slave side is

$$M_s s^2 E + C_s E = F_e \qquad (7.13)$$

where $E = X_m - X_s$ and $C_s = k_{ds}s + k_{ps}$. Obtaining a similar equation for the master side and subtracting (7.13) from it gives:

$$(M_m - M_s)s^2 E + (C_m - C_s)E = F_h - F_e \qquad (7.14)$$

In the ideal case $F_h = F_e$, hence

$$s^2 E + \frac{C_m - C_s}{M_m - M_s} E = 0 \qquad (7.15)$$

If we assume $(C_m - C_s)/(M_m - M_s) = C$ is a PD controller to ensure asymptotic convergence of $e(t)$ to zero, then we can simply choose the master and the slave PD controllers as $C_m = M_m C$ and $C_s = M_s C$, resulting in:

$$C_m/M_m = C_s/M_s \qquad (7.16)$$

Based on (7.16), the slave-side PD controller is tuned for tracking under the free motion condition, and the master-side controller will be a scaled version of that. The ultimate goal of tuning in a bilateral teleoperation system is to make the slave controller as "stiff" as possible, while keeping the master as "compliant" as possible. However, by making the slave controller stiff through increasing its gains, according to (7.16), the outputs of the master and the slave controllers can saturate causing high-frequency vibrations in the system. On the other hand, excessive reduction of the slave controller gains will cause underdamped (and low-frequency oscillatory) response. In practice, it was observed that for the haptic teleoperation system that we used in our experiments the range of the slave controller's gains for which saturation of the master and the slave controllers are avoided corresponds to a dominant pole location that leads to a very compliant and underdamped slave.

7.3.2 *Hybrid-type configurations*

Hybrid-type configurations of teleoperation systems do not have the tuning problems of admittance-type configurations. Figure 7.4 shows filtered

HPEB and HKFB teleoperation systems. Due to the asymmetric nature of the corresponding scattering matrices, stability analysis of neither of these configurations is mathematically tractable based on Theorem 5.4, as was the case with the symmetric networks. In their pioneering work on passivity-based time delay compensation in a bilateral teleoperation system, Anderson and Spong introduced the HPEB teleoperation configuration and based their proof of stability on modeling this system as a cascade of passive two-port networks [3]. This approach uses the fact that the cascade interconnection of any two passive systems is passive. The problem with the cited approach is that it cannot be extended to the case of an HKFB teleoperation system in a straightforward manner. A rigorous stability study of the HKFB architecture needs more developments and is beyond the scope of this discussion.

It is worth mentioning that the HKFB architecture possesses a scattering matrix, which is neither symmetric nor reciprocal implying that, although sufficient, passivityis not a necessary condition for its stability. The interest in passivity of a teleoperation system stems from the fact that it ensures absolutely stable performance for a class of multivariable systems that cannot be easily subjected to other methods of stability analysis, usually at the cost of performance.In practice, it was observed that by utilizing two additional lowpass filters in the system, one for filtering the measured slave/environment interaction force f_e before feeding it to the slave-side wave transformer and the other for filtering the reflected force f_{md} before applying it to the master robot, according to Figure 7.4b, it is possible to have better loop-shaping flexibility in order to obtain the best stable performance in the teleoperation system. It can be shown that even in the absence of any force sensor noise, these low-pass filters help to improve transparency by pushing the maximum singular values of the scattering matrix of the HKFB teleoperation system towards unity. The precise tuning of these filters depends on the characteristic of the force sensor and is basically an implementation issue.

7.4   4-Channel Architecture

7.4.1   *Delay-free case*

As it was discussed in Section 5.2.2, Figure 7.5 depicts a general 4CH bilateral teleoperation architecture [79, 153]. The operator and environment exogenous forces F_h' and F_e' are inputs independent of teleoperation system

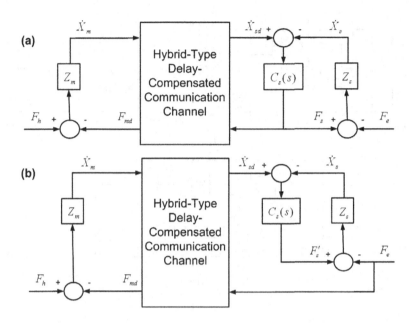

Fig. 7.4 Wave-based hybrid-type teleoperation systems: (a) HPEB; (b) HKFB.

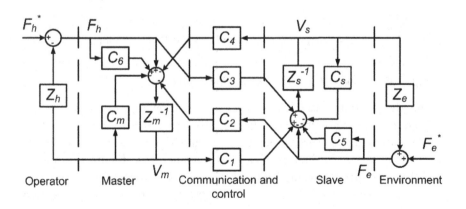

Fig. 7.5 4CH bilateral teleoperation system without time delay.

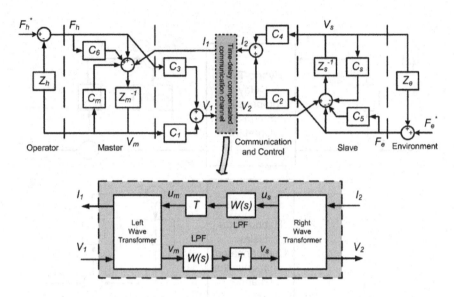

Fig. 7.6   Wave-based 4CH teleoperation system.

behavior.

The following ideal transparency condition set was derived for the 4CH architecture in Section 5.2.2:

$$C_1 = Z_{ts} \quad C_2 = 1 + C_6 \quad C_3 = 1 + C_5 \quad C_4 = -Z_{tm} \qquad (7.17)$$

where $Z_{tm} = M_m s + C_m(s) = M_m s + k_{dm} + k_{pm}/s$ and $Z_{ts} = M_s s + C_s(s) = M_s s + k_{ds} + k_{ps}/s$, assuming C_m and C_s to be PD controllers.

7.4.2   *Wave-based 4-channel architecture*

So far the passivity-based time delay compensation approach has been applied only to 2CH architectures. In order to extend this approach to a 4CH teleoperation architecture, we need to segregate the communication channel part of the system in Figure 7.5 as a two-port network. Figure 7.6 shows a possible method for accomplishing this extension. The non-physical input effort and flow pair for this two-port network model of the communication channel in Figure 7.6 are

$$V_1 = C_3 F_h + C_1 \dot{X}_m$$
$$I_2 = C_2 F_e + C_4 \dot{X}_s \qquad (7.18)$$

The master and the slave closed-loop equations can be written as:

$$\dot{X}_m Z_m = -\dot{X}_m C_m + F_h(1 + C_6) - I_1$$
$$\dot{X}_s Z_s = -\dot{X}_s C_s - F_e(1 + C_5) + V_2 \tag{7.19}$$

Therefore, the non-physical output flow and effort pair are

$$I_1 = F_h(1 + C_6) - \dot{X}_m Z_{tm}$$
$$V_2 = F_e(1 + C_5) + \dot{X}_s Z_{ts} \tag{7.20}$$

The communication channel effort and flow relationships in (7.18) and (7.20), from which input and output pseudo-power functions are calculated, are not unique but in their presented form they are independent of knowledge of Z_e and Z_h, which is an advantage for implementation. The communication channel can be modelled based on its inputs and outputs as

$$\begin{bmatrix} -I_1 \\ V_2 \end{bmatrix} = \begin{bmatrix} c_{11} & c_{12} \\ c_{21} & c_{22} \end{bmatrix} \begin{bmatrix} V_1 \\ I_2 \end{bmatrix} = C(s) \begin{bmatrix} V_1 \\ I_2 \end{bmatrix} \tag{7.21}$$

where the matrix C can be defined with respect to the hybrid matrix of the communication channel as

$$C(s) = H_{ch}^{-1}(s) \tag{7.22}$$

Using equation (7.21) in (7.19), the overall system can be represented by the following equations:

$$\dot{X}_m Z_{tm} = F_h(1 + C_6) + c_{11}V_1 + c_{12}I_2$$
$$\dot{X}_s Z_{ts} = -F_e(1 + C_5) + c_{21}V_1 + c_{22}I_2 \tag{7.23}$$

The outputs of the wave transformation block at the master side are

$$I_1 = \frac{\sqrt{2b}u_m - V_1}{b} \quad v_m = \frac{bu_m - \sqrt{2b}V_1}{b} \tag{7.24}$$

and at the slave side

$$V_2 = bI_2 - \sqrt{2b}v_s \quad u_s = \sqrt{2b}I_2 - v_s \tag{7.25}$$

Transformation (7.24) can be derived from the basic definition of wave variables (i.e., (7.6)) by taking the flow variable (I_1) and v_m as outputs and the effort variable (V_1) and u_m as inputs. Similarly, wave transformation (7.25) is obtained through selecting V_2 and u_s as outputs and I_2 and v_s as inputs. Wave variables v_m and u_s experience time delay T while passing through the communication channel in opposite directions. It can be easily checked that for the case of $T = 0$, $V_1 = V_2$ and $I_1 = I_2$, thus the original system of Figure 7.5 is recovered.

The input/output arrangement in (7.24) and (7.25) is due to the fact that the input/output relationship for the communication channel of the proposed 4CH architecture corresponds to an "inverse hybrid" representation of a two-port network (i.e., its inputs are V_1 and I_2 and its outputs are $-I_1$ and V_2, where the directions of the input and output flows corresponds to the convention set in [3]) – see equation (7.22), whereas that relationship is in the form of a hybrid model for the 2CH architecture of Figure 7.1.

7.4.3 *Transparency considerations*

Applying the condition set (7.17) for ideal transparency without time delay, the overall hybrid parameters of the proposed wave-based 4CH teleoperation system in Figure 7.6 are given by:

$$h_{11} = [(W^2 e^{-2sT} - 1)(Z_{ts}^2 - b^2 Z_{tm}^2)]/D_2$$
$$h_{12} = 2bW e^{-sT}(Z_{tm}C_3 + Z_{ts}C_2)/D_2$$
$$h_{21} = -2bW e^{-sT}(Z_{tm}C_3 + Z_{ts}C_2)/D_2$$
$$h_{22} = [(W^2 e^{-2sT} - 1)(b^2 C_2^2 - C_3^2)]/D_2 \tag{7.26}$$

where

$$D_2 = b(W^2 e^{-2sT} + 1)(Z_{ts}C_2 + Z_{tm}C_3)$$
$$+ (W^2 e^{-2sT} - 1)(-b^2 C_2 Z_{tm} - C_3 Z_{ts}) \tag{7.27}$$

The controller gains should be chosen in accordance with

$$C_s/C_m = M_s/M_m \tag{7.28}$$

as the master and the slave control actions need to be proportional to their inertias. This will ensure that the master and the slave have similar closed-loop behavior. Using (7.28), it can be easily shown that $Z_{ts}/Z_{tm} = M_s/M_m$. Setting h_{11} from (7.26) equal to zero under the ideal transparency condition according to (7.2) gives:

$$b_{ideal} = Z_{ts}/Z_{tm} \tag{7.29}$$

Similarly, for h_{22} to be equal to zero, we should have

$$C_3/C_2 = b_{ideal} \tag{7.30}$$

Using (7.29) and (7.30) in (7.26), expressions for h_{12} and h_{21} under ideal transparency condition can be derived as:

$$h_{12} = -h_{21} = W(s)e^{-sT} \qquad (7.31)$$

Equation (7.31) means that for $W(s) = 1$, the condition set (7.17) along with equations (7.29) and (7.30) are delayed ideal transparency provisions for the proposed 4CH architecture of Figure 7.6.

It can be shown that a teleoperation system represented by the delayed ideally transparent hybrid matrix in (7.2) cannot preserve passivity [3]. Therefore, a stability study in this case also needs to factor Z_h and Z_e. For the teleoperation system under ideal transparency conditions, if Z_{ts} is Hurwitz ($k_{ds}, k_{ps} > 0$), the input admittance transfer function based on the input F'_h and the output $\dot{X}_m$ can be simplified to

$$Y_{\text{in}} = (Z_h + Z_e e^{-2sT})^{-1} \qquad (7.32)$$

In order to present a descriptive stability analysis of an ideally transparent delayed teleoperation system, it is possible to use Padé approximation to simplify the characteristic polynomial in (7.32) and apply the Routh-Hurwitz criterion assuming $Z_h = (M_h s^2 + k_{dh}s + k_{ph})/s$ and $Z_e = k_{pe}/s$. For mathematical tractability, we use a first-order Padé approximation $e^{-2sT} \simeq (1 - sT)/(1 + sT)$ to re-write the characteristic equation in (7.32) as

$$M_h T s^3 + (k_{dh}T + M_h)s^2 +$$
$$(-k_{ph}\alpha T + k_{ph}T + k_{dh})s + k_{ph}\alpha + k_{ph} = 0 \qquad (7.33)$$

where $\alpha = k_{pe}/k_{pm}$. Applying the Routh-Hurwitz criterion to (7.33), the following condition on α as the necessary and sufficient condition for stability of the system represented by (7.32) can be derived

$$\alpha = \frac{k_{pe}}{k_{ph}} < \frac{k_{dh}(M_h + k_{dh}T + k_{ph}T^2)}{k_{ph}(2M_h + k_{dh}T)T} \qquad (7.34)$$

Equation (7.34) sets an upper bound on the remote environment stiffness k_{pe} depending on the operator parameters and time delay. Generally speaking, condition (7.34) is easy to meet particularly under small delays or with compliant environments, or through operator's adaptation to the remote environment characteristics.

7.4.4   3-channel architecture

As it was discussed in Section 5.2.2.3, another advantage of the general 4CH architecture of Figure 7.5 is that by proper adjustment of the local feedback parameters, it is possible to obtain two classes of 3CH control architectures, which can be transparent under ideal conditions [52]. The first class of 3CH architectures is derived by setting $C_2 = 1$ and $C_3 = 0$. As a consequence, $C_5 = -1$ and $C_6 = 0$. The second class of 3CH architectures is obtained by setting $C_2 = 0$ and $C_3 = 1$.

Deriving a wave-based 3CH architecture from the proposed wave-based 4CH architecture under ideal transparency provisions only affects h_{22}. In order to explain this further, assume under condition set (7.17) and provisions (7.28) and (7.29) that only the slave unity local force feedback is used (i.e., $C_5 = -1$ and $C_6 = 0$). It can be easily shown that h_{11}, h_{12}, and h_{21} still keep their ideal transparency values after this rearrangement. However, the new h_{22} is

$$h_{22} = (W^2 e^{-2sT} - 1)/(2Z_{tm}) \qquad (7.35)$$

According to (7.35), the bigger the magnitude of Z_{tm}, the closer h_{22} is to its ideal value of zero. This result suggests that this 3CH architecture is suitable for applications in which the master is heavy. On the other hand, if only the master unity local force feedback is used (i.e., $C_6 = -1$ and $C_5 = 0$), while h_{11}, h_{12}, and h_{21} remain unchanged from their ideal transparency values, the new h_{22} is given by

$$h_{22} = (1 - W^2 e^{-2sT})/(2Z_{ts}) \qquad (7.36)$$

which shows that the second 3CH architecture is suitable for applications with a heavy slave robot.

7.5   Experimental Performance Evaluation

For experimental performance evaluation, we used the force-reflective master-slave system described in Section 5.3.1 (see Figure 5.6). Recall that in the haptic interface, the friction/gravity effects are compensated for. Also, the master and the slave effective inertias are $M_m = 5.968 \times 10^{-4}$ kgm^2 and $M_s = 9.814 \times 10^{-3}$ kgm^2, respectively. In the experiments in this chapter, the master and slave subsystems were constrained for force-reflective teleoperation in the twist direction only (i.e. rotations about the instrument axis). The user twists the master back and forth causing the slave

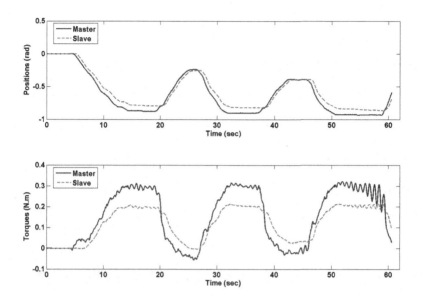

Fig. 7.7 Position and force tracking profiles for the 2CH position error based (PEB) teleoperation architecture with a round-trip delay of 200 ms.

to repeatedly probe a soft tissue (foam) phantom using a small rigid beam attached to the slave's end-effector for about 60 seconds. The instrument interactions with the tissue are measured and reflected in real-time to the user.

Figure 7.7 shows the master and the slave position and torque tracking profiles for a PEB teleoperation architecture with $b = 1$, $T = 100$ ms, $k_d = 3$, $k_p = 10$, and $f_{cut} = 5$ Hz. Assuming that a dedicated communication network is used, our choice of one-way time delay of 100 ms is approximately equal to the coast-to-coast communication delay in North America. Figure 7.8 illustrates the same tracking profiles for a modified direct force reflection teleoperation architecture with similar parameters, where the cut-off frequency for f_e and f_{md} first-order filters is 2 Hz. As can be deduced from these figures, the position tracking performance for the two systems are close to each other. However, the modified direct force reflection teleoperation system displays a superior force tracking performance, which demonstrates a higher level of transparency. This deduction is in accordance with the results presented in [2] for teleoperation systems without time delay.

To further investigate the relative transparency of these two systems, a

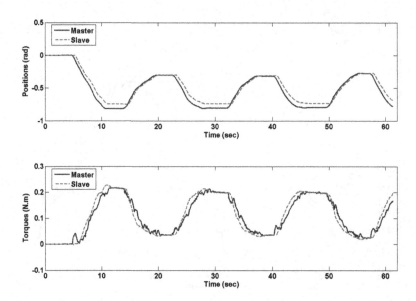

Fig. 7.8   Position and force tracking profiles for the 2CH direct force reflection (DFR) teleoperation architecture with a round-trip delay of 200 ms.

second set of free-motion tests was performed, which in conjunction with the previous contact-mode tests, can be used to determine the hybrid parameters of the teleoperation system in the frequency domain. The magnitudes of the hybrid parameters of the 2CH PEB and direct force reflection teleoperation architectures for $T = 100$ ms are shown in Figure 7.9. Due to the human operator's limited input bandwidth, these identified hybrid parameters can be considered valid up to a frequency of 60 rad/s.

Figure 7.9 is an indication of the superiority of the direct force reflection architecture in terms of transparent performance considering the ideal transparency requirements in the presence of a communication channel time delay, as specified by (7.2). The hybrid parameter $h_{11} = F_h/X_m|_{F_e=0}$ is the input impedance in free-motion condition. High values of h_{11} for position error-based architecture are evidence of the fact that even when the slave is in free space, the user will feel some force as a result of any control inaccuracies (i.e., nonzero position errors), thus giving a "sticky" feel of free-motion movements. On the other hand, since the direct force reflection architecture uses f_e measurements, its input impedance in free-motion condition will be significantly lower making the feeling of free space much more realistic. The parameter $h_{12} = F_h/F_e|_{X_m=0}$ is a measure of force tracking for

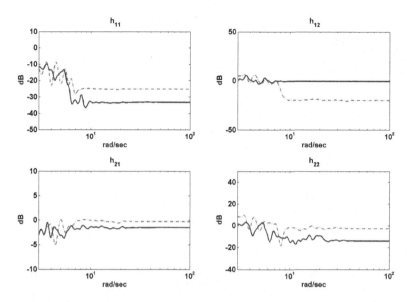

Fig. 7.9   Magnitudes of the hybrid parameters for the PEB and DFR architectures with a round-trip delay of 200 ms (dashed: PEB; solid: DFR).

the haptic teleoperation system. The better force tracking performance of direct force reflection architecture in Figure 7.9, i.e., $h_{12} \approx 0$ dB, confirms the time-domain results observed in Figures 7.7 and 7.8. The parameter $h_{21} = -X_s/X_m|_{F_e=0}$ is a measure of the position tracking performance. In this respect, the spectrum of the PEB architecture is a little closer to 0 dB, which is indicative of a slightly better position tracking performance. It is worthwhile mentioning that because of the finite stiffness of the slave and also the backlash present in the slave's gearhead, the accuracy of $h_{22} = -X_s/F_e|_{X_m=0}$ estimates is less than that of the rest of the hybrid parameters.

As can be seen in Figure 7.7, with the PEB architecture, there are vibrations in the master and slave positions and forces in the contact mode. It was also observed that the magnitudes of these vibrations increase with time delay. While stability in the wave-based time delay compensation approach is guaranteed in theory regardless of the time delay, in practice and consistent with previous studies [3, 101], such vibrations exist and may be due to implementation reasons such as discretization or limited controller bandwidth. As can be seen in Figure 7.9, these vibrations affect the h_{12} parameter of the PEB teleoperation architecture. However, as shown in

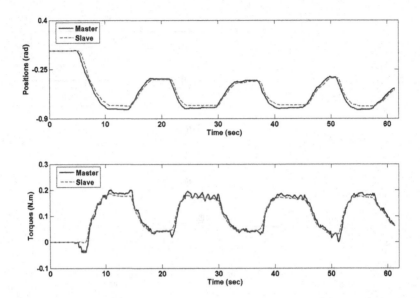

Fig. 7.10   Position and force tracking profiles for the wave-based 4CH teleoperation architecture with a round-trip delay of 200 ms.

the force profile of Figure 7.8 and the h_{12} spectrum of Figure 7.9, force tracking is much less subjected to unwanted vibrations in the case of the direct force reflection architecture. These results are indicative of the fact that transparency is improved by providing slave force sensor data to the bilateral control algorithm.

Figure 7.10 shows the master and the slave positions and torque tracking profiles for a 4CH wave-based architecture based on the ideal transparency criteria (7.17), (7.29), and (7.30) with single-way time delay $T = 100$ ms, $C_2 = C_3 = 0.5$, $b = 8$, $C_m = 40M_m(10 + s)$ (PD position controller), $C_s = 40M_s(10 + s)$, and $f_{cut} = 1$ Hz. Figure 7.11 shows the same results for an 3CH wave-base architecture with only the unity local force feedback at the slave side (no master local force feedback). All the other parameters are identical. The reason for choosing this type of 3CH architecture is that in our setup, the slave manipulator is sensorized to measure its interaction force with the environment, while in the absence of a force sensor the master uses a system observer for contact force estimation. The results in these two figures indicate that the 3CH architecture is better suited for our setup in comparison with the 4CH architecture.

The magnitudes of the hybrid parameters of the wave-based 4CH and

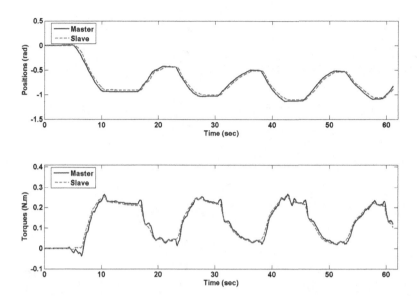

Fig. 7.11 Position and force tracking profiles for the wave-based 3CH teleoperation architecture with a round-trip delay of 200 ms.

3CH teleoperation architectures are shown in Figure 7.12. The force and position tracking performances (reflected in the h_{12} and h_{21} spectra of Figure 7.12) in the case of the 3CH architecture is almost perfect. The superiority of performance in the case of the 3CH architecture can be attributed to the higher gain of the slave local feedback, which allows for a lower level of master force feedforward and consequently, less contribution from the master side force observer. Unlike the case of the 2CH position error based architecture, 4CH and 3CH architectures do not show any sign of vibrations under contact conditions.

In terms of transparency, 3CH architecture can be considered the best among the four teleoperation control architectures under study. Direct force reflection is showing very good transparency, bearing in mind that it only needs the minimum requirement in terms of the communication channel bandwidth. Also, considering the fact that 3CH and 4CH architectures work under ideal transparency conditions (7.17), (7.29), and (7.30), they are more sensitive to system parameter variations in comparison to a less transparent architecture such as the 2CH direct force reflection. With respect to position tracking under contact conditions, which is not reflected in any of the hybrid parameter spectra, it can be concluded from Figures 7.7,

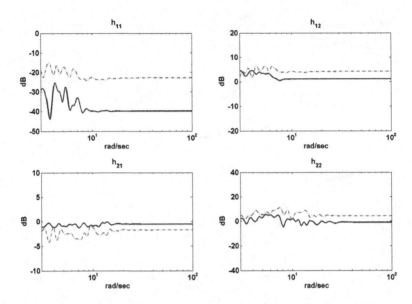

Fig. 7.12   Magnitudes of the hybrid parameters for the wave-based 4CH and 3CH architectures with a round-trip delay of 200 ms (dashed: 4CH; solid: 3CH).

7.8, 7.10, and 7.11 that the 3CH and 4CH architectures outperform both of the 2CH architectures. This can be attributed to the fact that the 2CH architectures use only one PD controller at the master side, while a 4CH architecture has a second position controller at the master side. The role of this controller becomes more pronounced when F_e is non-zero.

7.6   Concluding Remarks

In this chapter, we quantitatively compared the performance of two different approaches for wave-based time-delay compensation in a master-slave system. The first approach is based upon the traditional 2-channel bilateral wave-based teleoperation control architecture, in which the system is made robust against communication channel latencies through the introduction of wave transformers. We have effectively improved the transparency of this system by making use of force measurements at the slave side without imposing additional costs on the stability of the system. In the second approach, we have extended the use of wave theory for time-delay compensation to a 4-channel teleoperation control architecture. This control architecture is capable of achieving ideal transparency under delay-free conditions, and we have shown that ideal transparency can also be maintained in our proposed 4-channel wave-based architecture for teleoperation under delay.

Appendix A

Mechanical Description of the Slave

The slave subsystem is shown in Figure A.1. It consists of

- The base 1-1 and the fulcrum 1-2.
- The laparoscopic instrument assembly 2.
- The motor and encoder for the roll direction 3-1.
- The 2-DOF gimbals assembly 3.
- The PHANToM 1.5A haptic device 4.

A.1 Fulcrum

The base and the fulcrum for the slave are similar to the master's base and fulcrum in Appendix B. The fulcrum, through which the laparoscopic instrument is inserted, is co-located with the incision made on the patient's body. The fulcrum 1-2 is a 4-DOF gimbals assembly allowing motions in roll, pitch, yaw and insertion directions. A potentiometer mounted on the fulcrum measures the pitch angle for measurement redundancy purposes.

A.2 Laparoscopic instrument assembly

The laparoscopic instrument assembly 2 is passed through the fulcrum. It consists of the instrument shaft 2-1, the tip actuation mechanism and force/torque sensors.

A.3   The motor and encoder for the roll direction

A geared motor and encoder connects the laparoscopic instrument assembly 2 to the 2-DOF gimbals 3. The motor turns the laparoscopic instrument sub-assembly to replicate user hand's rotations on the master side.

A.4   2-DOF gimbals assembly

The 2-DOF gimbals 3 is comprised of two arcuate arms and a brace that holds onto the motor and encoder sub-assembly 3-1 and is attached to the end-point of the PHANToM haptic device 4. If the motor and encoder sub-assembly faces resistance while trying to rotate the laparoscopic instrument and the tissue grasped by the tip, the gimbals assembly will not twist into itself. This is because the main axis of the motor and encoder sub-assembly and the axis of a revolute joint connecting the two arcuate arms in the 2-DOF gimbals are never parallel within the device workspace.

A.5   PHANToM haptic device

The PHANToM device 4 is integrated into the slave subsystem for simplicity. The PHANToM can be positioned in front of the base 1-1 or on its side, in order to provide optimal workspace and manipulability of the laparoscopic instrument. Figure A.1 shows only a simplified drawing of the PHANToM device.

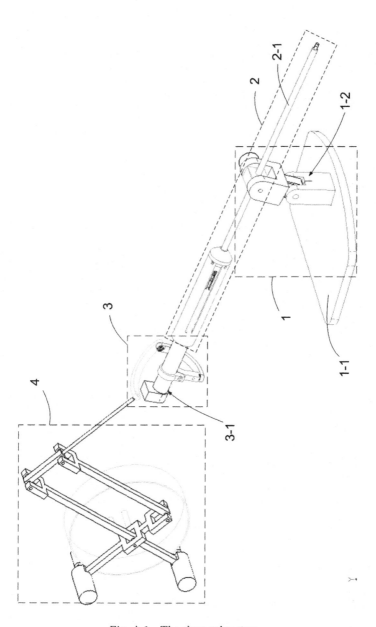

Fig. A.1 The slave subsystem.

Appendix B

Mechanical Description of the Master

The master subsystem, which provides haptic feedback to the user, is shown in Figure B.1. It comprises

- The base 1-1 and the fulcrum 1-2.
- The instrument shaft 2 passing through fulcrum.
- The force-reflecting finger loops assembly 3.
- The assembly for force reflection in the roll direction 4.
- The PHANToM 1.5A haptic device 5.

B.1 Fulcrum

The fulcrum 1-2 shown in Figure B.2 realizes a virtual incision point through which the instrument is inserted into the body. The fulcrum is a 4-DOF gimbals assembly allowing motions in roll, pitch, yaw and insertion directions. While these three angles and the displacement can be found based on measurements from the rest of the master subsystem, a potentiometer is mounted on the gimbals for redundancy in measurements.

B.2 Instrument shaft

As shown in Figure B.1, the shaft 2 acts as the endoscopic instrument and is passed through the opening of the fulcrum.

B.3   Force-reflecting finger loops

The force reflecting finger loops 3 shown in Figure B.3 is a 1-DOF haptic mechanism attached to one end of the shaft 2. The pre-tensioned cable pinned at the two ends of the sector disk and wrapped several times around the motor pulley provides power transmission. The motor is secured to a fixed handle and turns the other handle through the aforementioned cable transmission. The motor has an encoder to measure the angle of the finger loops relative to one another. The sector disk and the handle fixed to the sector disk apply a force against the squeezing face of the user's thumb.

B.4   Force reflection in the roll direction

Two views of the 1-DOF assembly for force reflection in the roll direction are depicted in Figure B.4. The pre-tensioned cable is pinned to disk at 0° and 360° and wrapped several times around the motor pulley in order to provide power transmission. The disk is fixed to the distal end of the shaft (see Figure B.1) while the motor is secured to a joint, which connects the end point of the PHANToM to the distal end of shaft. Thus, the motor turns the shaft through the cable transmission described above, resulting in the application of a torque on the wrist of the user. The joint shown in Figure B.4 includes an encoder for measuring pitch motion and an encoder for measuring yaw motion of the instrument. Also, the motor encoder measures the roll angle of the shaft.

B.5   PHANToM haptic device

In Figure B.1, a PHANToM 1.5A haptic device is built into the master interface. This haptic device provides six degrees of freedom input control, only three of which are active (i.e., with force reflection). The PHANToM can be oriented normally or upside down and positioned in front of the base or on its side, in order to provide optimal dexterity and comfort for the user. Figure B.1 shows only a simplified drawing of the PHANToM haptic device.

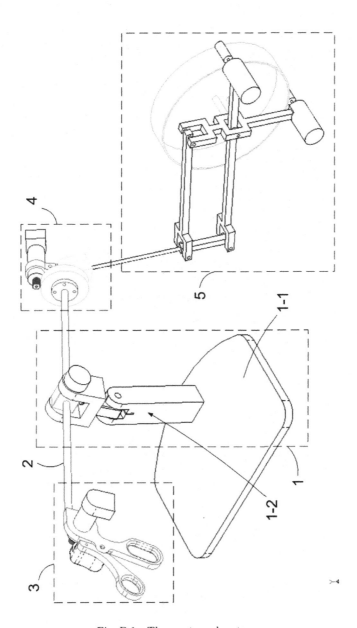

Fig. B.1   The master subsystem.

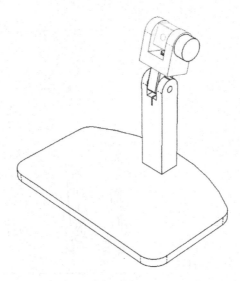

Fig. B.2   The base and the fulcrum.

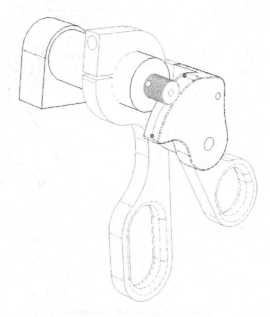

Fig. B.3   The force-reflecting finger loops.

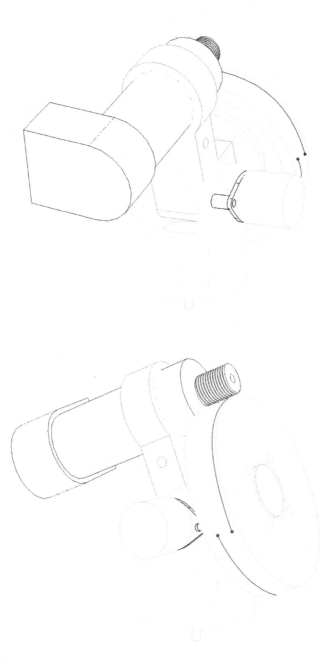

Fig. B.4   Two views of the mechanism for force reflection in the roll direction.

Appendix C

Kinematics and Dynamics of the PHANToM Haptic Device

The PHANToM haptic interface is a robot in which the position of its endpoint is measured with respect to a home position. The home position is where all control surfaces are at their right angle positions, i.e., where the arms and motors are at right angles to one another (see Figure C.1). In this appendix, the kinematics and dynamics of the PHANToM model 1.5A are presented [19]. We will use the variables and parameters shown in Figure C.1.

C.1 Forward kinematics

The forward kinematics mapping $g_{st}(\theta)$ is given in the following closed form:

$$
\begin{pmatrix}
\cos(\theta_1) & -\sin(\theta_1)\sin(\theta_3) & \cos(\theta_3)\sin(\theta_1) & \sin(\theta_1)(\ell_1\cos(\theta_2) + \ell_2\sin(\theta_3)) \\
0 & \cos(\theta_3) & \sin(\theta_3) & \ell_2 - \ell_2\cos(\theta_3) + \ell_1\sin(\theta_2) \\
-\sin(\theta_1) & -\cos(\theta_1)\sin(\theta_3) & \cos(\theta_1)\cos(\theta_3) & -\ell_1 + \cos(\theta_1)(\ell_1\cos(\theta_2) + \ell_2 sin(\theta_3)) \\
0 & 0 & 0 & 1
\end{pmatrix}
$$

$$(C.1)$$

C.2 Inverse kinematics

As a 3-DOF manipulator, the inverse kinematics problem is to find the set of joint angles $(\theta_1, \theta_2, \theta_3)$ corresponding to the end-effector position (x_0, y_0, z_0). The following equations meet the above requirement:

$$\theta_1 = \text{atan2}(x_0, z_0 + \ell_1) \tag{C.2}$$

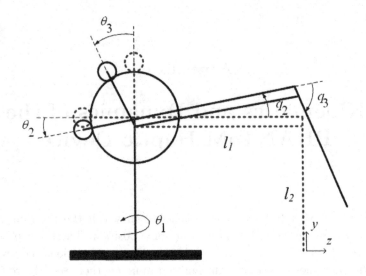

Fig. C.1   The PHANToM manipulator. Dashed lines show the home configuration.

$$\theta_2 = \text{atan2}(y_0 - \ell_2, R) + \cos^{-1}\left(\frac{\ell_1^2 + r^2 - \ell_2^2}{2\ell_1 r}\right) \tag{C.3}$$

$$\theta_3 = \theta_2 + \cos^{-1}\left(\frac{\ell_1^2 + r^2 - \ell_2^2}{2\ell_1 \ell_2}\right) - \frac{\pi}{2} \tag{C.4}$$

where

$$R = \sqrt{x_0^2 + (z_0 + \ell_1)^2} \tag{C.5}$$

$$r = \sqrt{x_0^2 + (y_0 - \ell_2)^2 + (z_0 + \ell_1)^2} \tag{C.6}$$

C.3   Manipulator Jacobian

Spatial and body Jacobians of the manipulator are respectively given by

$$J^s(\theta) = \begin{pmatrix} \ell_1 & -\ell_1 \sin(\theta_1)\sin(\theta_2) & \sin(\theta_1)(\ell_2 + \ell_1 \sin(\theta_2)) \\ 0 & \ell_1 \cos(\theta_2) & \ell_1(\cos(\theta_1) - \cos(\theta_2)) \\ 0 & -\ell_1 \cos(\theta_1)\sin(\theta_2) & \cos(\theta_1)(\ell_2 + \ell_1 \sin(\theta_2)) \\ 0 & 0 & -\cos(\theta_2) \\ 1 & 0 & 0 \\ 0 & 0 & \sin(\theta_1) \end{pmatrix} \tag{C.7}$$

$$J^b(\theta) = \begin{pmatrix} \ell_1\cos(\theta_2) + \ell_2\sin(\theta_3) & 0 & 0 \\ 0 & \ell_1\cos(\theta_2 - \theta_3) & 0 \\ 0 & -\ell_1\sin(\theta_2 - \theta_3) & \ell_2 \\ 0 & 0 & -1 \\ \cos(\theta_3) & 0 & 0 \\ \sin(\theta_3) & 0 & 0 \end{pmatrix} \quad (C.8)$$

C.4 Dynamics

Lagrangian formulation can be used to derive the dynamic equations of the manipulator. Once the Lagrangian L is found, the system equations of motion can be calculated as

$$\frac{d}{dt}\frac{\partial L}{\partial \dot{\theta}_i} - \frac{\partial L}{\partial \theta_i} = \tau_i, \quad , i = 1, 2, 3. \quad (C.9)$$

In closed form, we have

$$\begin{pmatrix} M_{11} & 0 & 0 \\ 0 & M_{22} & M_{23} \\ 0 & M_{32} & M_{33} \end{pmatrix} \begin{pmatrix} \ddot{\theta}_1 \\ \ddot{\theta}_2 \\ \ddot{\theta}_3 \end{pmatrix} \begin{pmatrix} C_{11} & C_{12} & C_{13} \\ C_{21} & 0 & C_{23} \\ C_{31} & C_{32} & 0 \end{pmatrix} \begin{pmatrix} \dot{\theta}_1 \\ \dot{\theta}_2 \\ \dot{\theta}_3 \end{pmatrix} + \begin{pmatrix} 0 \\ N_2 \\ N_3 \end{pmatrix} = \begin{pmatrix} \tau_1 \\ \tau_2 \\ \tau_3 \end{pmatrix} \quad (C.10)$$

where

$$M_{11} = \frac{1}{8}(4I_{ayy} + 4I_{azz} + 8I_{baseyy} + 4I_{beyy} + 4I_{bezz} + 4I_{cyy} + 4I_{czz} + 4I_{dfyy}$$

$$+ 4I_{dfzz} + 4\ell_1^2 m_a + \ell_2^2 m_a + \ell_1^2 m_c + 4\ell_3^2 m_c) + \frac{1}{8}(4I_{beyy} - 4I_{bezz} + 4I_{cyy}$$

$$- 4I_{czz} + \ell_1^2(4m_a + m_c))\cos(2\theta_2) + \frac{1}{8}(4I_{ayy} - 4I_{azz} + 4I_{dfyy} - 4I_{dfzz}$$

$$- \ell_2^2 m_a - 4\ell_3^2 m_c)\cos(2\theta_3) + \ell_1(\ell_2 m_a + \ell_3 m_c)\cos(\theta_2)\sin(\theta_3)$$

$$M_{22} = \frac{1}{4}(4(I_{bexx} + I_{cxx} + \ell_1^2 m_a) + \ell_1^2 m_c)$$

$$M_{23} = -\frac{1}{2}\ell_1(\ell_2 m_a + \ell_3 m_c)\sin(\theta_2 - \theta_3)$$

$$M_{32} = -\frac{1}{2}\ell_1(\ell_2 m_a + \ell_3 m_c)\sin(\theta_2 - \theta_3)$$

$$M_{33} = \frac{1}{4}(4I_{axx} + 4I_{dfxx} + \ell_2^2 m_a + 4\ell_3^2 m_c)$$

and

$$C_{11} = \frac{1}{8}(-2\sin(\theta_2)((4I_{beyy} - 4I_{bezz} + 4I_{cyy} - 4I_{czz} + 4\ell_1^2 m_a + \ell_1^2 m_c)\cos(\theta_2)$$

$$+ 2\ell_1(\ell_2 m_a + \ell_3 m_c)\sin(\theta_3))\dot{\theta}_2 + 2\cos(\theta_3)(2\ell_1(\ell_2 m_a + \ell_3 m_c)\cos(\theta_2) + (-4I_a$$
$$+ 4I_{azz} - 4I_{dfyy} + 4I_{dfzz} + \ell_2^2 m_a + 4\ell_3^2 m_c)\sin(\theta_3))\dot{\theta}_3)$$

$$C_{12} = -\frac{1}{8}((4I_{beyy} - 4I_{bezz} + 4I_{cyy} - 4I_{czz} + \ell_1^2(4m_a + m_c))\sin(2\theta_2) + 4\ell_1(\ell_2 m_a$$
$$+ \ell_3 m_c)\sin(\theta_2)\sin(\theta_3))\dot{\theta}_1$$

$$C_{13} = -\frac{1}{8}(-4\ell_1(\ell_2 m_a + \ell_3 m_c)\cos(\theta_2)\cos(\theta_3) - (-4I_{ayy} + 4I_{azz} - 4I_{dfyy}$$
$$+ 4I_{dfzz} + \ell_2^2 m_a + 4\ell_3^2 m_c)\sin(2\theta_3))\dot{\theta}_1$$

$$C_{21} = -C_{12}$$

$$C_{23} = \frac{1}{2}\ell_1(\ell_2 m_a + \ell_3 m_c)\cos(\theta_2 - \theta_3)\dot{\theta}_3$$

$$C_{31} = -C_{13}$$

$$C_{32} = \frac{1}{2}\ell_1(\ell_2 m_a + \ell_3 m_c)\cos(\theta_2 - \theta_3)\dot{\theta}_2$$

$$N_2 = \frac{1}{2}g(2\ell_1 m_a + 2\ell_5 m_{be} + \ell_1 m_c)\cos(\theta_2)$$

$$N_3 = \frac{1}{2}g(\ell_2 m_a + 2\ell_3 m_c - 2\ell_6 m_{df})\sin(\theta_3)$$

Note that $M(\theta)$ is positive definite and $\dot{M}(\theta) - 2C(\theta, \dot{\theta})$ is skew symmetric. The numerical values of the parameters appearing above are as follows:

$\ell_1 = 0.215; \ell_2 = 0.170; \ell_3 = 0.0325; \ell_5 = 0.0368; \ell_6 = 0.0527;$

$m_a = 0.0202; m_c = 0.0249; m_{be} = 0.2359; m_{df} = 0.1906;$

$I_{axx} = 0.4864 \times 10^{-4}; I_{ayy} = 0.0018 \times 10^{-4}; I_{azz} = 0.4864 \times 10^{-4};$

$I_{cxx} = 0.959 \times 10^{-4}; I_{cyy} = 0.959 \times 10^{-4}; I_{czz} = 0.0051 \times 10^{-4};$

$I_{bexx} = 11.09 \times 10^{-4}; I_{beyy} = 10.06 \times 10^{-4}; I_{bezz} = 0.591 \times 10^{-4};$

$I_{dfxx} = 7.11 \times 10^{-4}; I_{dfyy} = 0.629 \times 10^{-4}; I_{dfzz} = 6.246 \times 10^{-4};$

$I_{baseyy} = 11.87 \times 10^{-4}; g = 9.81;$

Appendix D

1-DOF Master System Modeling and Identification

D.1 Dynamic modeling

The 1-DOF dynamic models of the master and the slave in the twist direction need to be determined in order to be able to implement the bilateral control laws discussed in Chapters 5 and 7. The dynamics of the 1-DOF master device excluding the friction terms can be written as

$$\tau_m = (m\ell^2 + I_{zz})\ddot{\theta}_m + mg\ell \sin(\theta_m + \alpha) \qquad (D.1)$$

where, as shown in Figure D.1, τ_m and θ_m are the joint torque and angular position at the motor output shaft, respectively. The center of mass m of the master is located at a distance ℓ and an angle α with respect to the master's axis of rotation. I_{zz} is the master's mass moment of inertia with respect to the axis of rotation.

To include the effect of friction in (D.1), consider two rigid bodies that make contact through (virtual) elastic bristles. The friction force/torque τ_{fric} between the two can be modeled based on their relative velocity $\dot{\theta}$ and the bristles's average deflection z as [28, 73]:

$$\frac{dz}{dt} = \dot{\theta} - \sigma_0 \frac{|\dot{\theta}|}{s(\dot{\theta})} z \qquad (D.2)$$

$$\tau_{\text{fric}} = \sigma_0 z + \sigma_1 \frac{dz}{dt} + \sigma\dot{\theta} \qquad (D.3)$$

where σ_0, σ_1 are the stiffness and damping parameters for the friction dynamics, and the term $\sigma\dot{\theta}$ accounts for viscous friction. A model of $s(\dot{\theta})$ that describes the Stribeck effect is given by $s(\dot{\theta}) = \tau_c(1-e^{-a|\dot{\theta}|})+\tau_s e^{-a|\dot{\theta}|}$ where τ_c and τ_s are Coulomb and stiction frictions, respectively. At steady state ($dz/dt = 0$), it follows from (D.2) that z approaches $z_{ss} = \text{sgn}(\dot{\theta})s(\dot{\theta})/\sigma_0$. Therefore, using (D.3), friction can be written as

$$\tau_{\text{fric}} = \sigma\dot{\theta} + \tau_c(1 - e^{-a|\dot{\theta}|})\text{sgn}(\dot{\theta}) + \tau_s e^{-a|\dot{\theta}|}\text{sgn}(\dot{\theta}) \qquad (D.4)$$

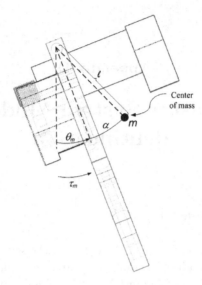

Fig. D.1   The master handle.

For the master device, assuming asymmetry in Stribeck friction effects when the master moves in the positive and negative directions, the dynamics can be written as

$$\tau_m = M_m \ddot{\theta}_m + G \sin(\theta_m + \alpha) + \sigma \dot{\theta}_m$$
$$+ \tau_{c_1}(1 - e^{-a_1|\dot{\theta}_m|})u_{\dot{\theta}_m} + \tau_{s_1}e^{-a_1|\dot{\theta}_m|}u_{\dot{\theta}_m}$$
$$+ \tau_{c_2}(1 - e^{-a_2|\dot{\theta}_m|})u_{-\dot{\theta}_m} + \tau_{s_2}e^{-a_2|\dot{\theta}_m|}u_{-\dot{\theta}_m} \qquad (D.5)$$

where τ_{c_i}, τ_{s_i} and a_i correspond to the positive direction ($\dot{\theta}_m > 0$) for $i = 1$ and to the negative direction ($\dot{\theta}_m < 0$) for $i = 2$, and $u(.)$ is the unity step function.

D.2   Parametric identification

The master dynamics (D.5) are unknown in terms of the rigid-body parameters for inertia and gravity M_m, G, α, and in the friction parameters σ, τ_{c_1}, τ_{s_1}, a_1, τ_{c_2}, τ_{s_2} and a_2. To identify these parameters, sinusoidal input torques $\tau_m = A\sin(2\pi ft)$ were applied to the master where the magnitudes and frequencies were chosen to cover various operating conditions of the system: $A \in \{0.03, 0.06, 0.09, 0.12, 0.15\}$ N.m and $f \in \{0.1, 0.5, 1\}$ Hz.

Table D.1   Identified master model parameters.

M_m	5.97×10^{-4}	kg.m^2
G	1.04×10^{-1}	N.m
α	9.3965	deg
σ	6.88×10^{-4}	N.m.sec/rad
τ_{c_1}	1.98×10^{-2}	N.m
τ_{s_1}	0	N.m
a_1	55.2	sec/rad
τ_{c_2}	-1.62×10^{-2}	N.m
τ_{s_2}	0	N.m
a_2	42.1	sec/rad

Moreover, experiments were performed with the summation of two sinusoidal signals as the input torque in order to increase the degree of persistence excitation of the input (the sum of n sinusoids is persistent excitation of an order no less than $2n - 2$ [124]). The resulting (τ_m, θ_m) pairs for all experiments were concatenated to form a complete set of input/output data. The joint position data were filtered by a 3rd-order Butterworth filter implemented using a zero-phase-distortion routine (Matlab function *filtfilt*) to remove the measurement noise. To find $\dot{\theta}_m$ for off-line system identification, the filtered position data were differentiated using the two-point central difference formula

$$\dot{y}(t) = \frac{y(t + T_s) - y(t - T_s)}{2T_s} \tag{D.6}$$

where T_s is the sampling time. Using the joint torque, position, velocity and acceleration data obtained above, a nonlinear multivariable minimization procedure (Matlab function *fminimax*) was used to find the parameter estimates that best fit the dynamic model (D.5). The identified parameters are listed in Table D.1. The above identified parameters were used to compensate for the gravity and friction effects, thus simplifying the dynamic model of the master to $\tau_m = M_m \ddot{\theta}_m$.

Appendix E

Virtual Reality Peripheral Network

The Virtual Reality Peripheral Network (VRPN) is an open-source library that provides a network-transparent and device-independent interface to virtual reality peripherals [138]. This means that:

- The application programs remain unaware of the network topology.
- All virtual reality (VR) peripheral devices with the same functionality are accessed using the same set of classes and methods. Therefore, no client-side change is needed when moving an application to different sets of VR devices.

The key idea in VRPN is factoring devices by function. Rather than providing drivers for a set of devices, VRPN offers interfaces for a set of functions. Each supported VR device[1] is factored into several interfaces each with a certain functionality, e.g., tracker, haptic device, button device, sound server, camera, etc. For instance, the VRPN server for a PHANToM device exports Tracker, ForceDevice and Button interfaces under the same device name and the client deals with the PHANToM as if it were three separate devices, one for each of its functions.

The VRPN library is compiled both on the client side and the server side. VRPN can run the client and the server on different machines, as different processes on the same machine, or within the same process. There is a generic server that reads a configuration file for instructions about which devices to open. On the client side, an application uses one or more VRPN devices by creating one or more VRPN application objects (e.g., vrpn_Tracker_Remote, vrpn_ForceDevice_Remote, vrpn_Button_Remote,

---

[1]Examples of the supported devices are Ascension Flock of Birds tracker, Sensable Technologies PHANToM haptic device, 5DT glove tracker, and Zaber Technologies linear positioning elements. For a complete list of the supported devices, see www.vrpn.org.

etc.). To open a PHANToM device connected to a machine with IP address
IP both as a Tracker and as a ForceDevice, the following would be done:

```
vrpn_Tracker_Remote myTracker("PHANToM@IP");
```

```
vrpn_ForceDevice_Remote myForceDevice("PHANToM@IP");
```

For object type `vrpn_Tracker_Remote`, the client-side application defines a callback function to the object that is called whenever a new data
value is received from the device. For `vrpn_ForceDevice _Remote`, the application calls member functions to provide commands to the remote device.
VRPN takes care of packaging the requests and sending them to the remote
device. VRPN also time stamps all messages to and from devices. Regardless of the object type, the application should call the object's `mainloop()`
member function once at each sampling time:

```
myTracker->mainloop();
```

```
myForceDevice->mainloop();
```

In the teleoperation system discussed in Chapters 2 and 3, three of
the five DOFs present in the master and the slave subsystems are provided by the PHANToM device integrated into each subsystem. Therefore,
while master-slave communication in these 3 DOFs is directly supported
by VRPN, it is necessary to use text messaging for communication in the
other two DOFs. VRPN supports sending text messages to communicate
human-readable information, warnings, and error messages. We use the
`vrpn_Connection` class to deliver messages locally and across network connections using callback handlers. For a connection to be set up, a listening
connection and a remote connection should be created. The sender creates the connections' listening endpoint, which will listen for requests on a
to-be-specified UDP (user datagram protocol) port, say port 4503:

```
vrpn_Connection *myServer = new vrpn_Connection(4503);
```

The `mainloop()` function of the above listening instance needs to be called
at each sampling time to check for incoming packets. The receiver creates
a device that sets up the remote endpoint by passing the complete name
of the device that is to be opened. For example, if the above sender was
created on a machine with IP address IP, the following is done:

```
vrpn_Connection *myReceiver =
        vrpn_get_connection_by_name("myServer@IP:4503");
```

The remote connection opens a TCP (transport control protocol) socket for listening and sends a UDP datagram to the specified port on the listening connection that tells it the machine name and port number of the TCP socket. In response to this, the listening connection establishes a TCP link to the remote connection. Then, each side of the connection opens a new UDP port and sends a description of the port to the other across the TCP channel. In this way, a path for low-latency and unreliable UDP-based traffic[2] to flow from the sender to the receiver is established. At this point, the connections describe to each other their local sender and message type information and the communication starts. Figure 5.7 in Chapter 5 shows what information is being sent and received through text messaging in the master-slave system.

---

[2]While TCP provides a point-to point channel for confirmation-based communication, UDP provides communication that is neither connection based nor confirmation based. In return, the Internet communication latencies are much lower and less fluctuating with UDP compared to TCP [96]. This makes UDP the protocol of choice for real-time control.

Appendix F

t-Test and ANOVA

The t-test is the most commonly used method to evaluate the differences in means between two groups. Theoretically, the t-test can be used even if the sample sizes are very small (e.g., as small as 10), as long as the variables are normally distributed within each group and the variation of scores in the two groups is not reliably different.

Given two paired sets x_i and y_i of n measured values, the paired t-test determines whether they differ from each other in a significant way under the assumptions that the paired differences are independent and identically normally distributed. The normality assumption can be evaluated by looking at the distribution of the data (via histograms) or by performing a normality test. The equality of variances assumption can be verified with the F-test. To apply t-test, let $\hat{x}_i = (x_i - \bar{x})$ and $\hat{y}_i = (y_i - \bar{y})$ where $\bar{x}$ and $\bar{y}$ are means the two paired sets; then t is defined by

$$t = (\bar{x} - \bar{y})\sqrt{\frac{n(n-1)}{\sum_{i=1}^{n}(\hat{x}_i - \hat{y}_i)^2}} \tag{F.1}$$

This statistic has $n - 1$ degrees of freedom. A table of Student's t-distribution confidence intervals can be used to determine the significance level at which two distributions differ. The corresponding p-value reported with a t-test represents the probability of error involved in accepting the research hypothesis about the existence of a difference. Technically speaking, this is the probability of error associated with rejecting the hypothesis of no difference between the two categories of observations (corresponding to the groups) in the population when, in fact, the hypothesis is true. Some researchers suggest that if the difference is in the predicted direction, it is possible to consider only one half (one "tail") of the probability distribution and thus divide the standard p-level reported with a t-test (a "two-tailed" probability) by two.

Similar to the two-sample t-test, "Analysis of Variance" (ANOVA) provides the means for testing hypotheses about the mean (average) of a dependent variable across different groups. In statistics, ANOVA is a collection of statistical models, and their associated procedures, in which the observed variance is partitioned into components due to different explanatory variables. While the t-test is used to compare the means between two groups, one-way ANOVA is used when the study involves three or more levels of a single independent variable. The ANOVA test procedure produces an F-test statistic, which is used to test the statistical significance of the differences among the obtained means of two or more random samples from a given population.

Bibliography

[1] Abolmaesumi, P., Salcudean, S. E., Zhu, W. H., Sirouspour, M. R. and Di-Maio, S. P. (2002). Image-guided control of a robot for medical ultrasound, *IEEE Transactions on Robotics and Automation* **18**, pp. 11–23.

[2] Aliaga, I., Rubio, A. and Sanchez, E. (2004). Experimental quantitative comparison of different control architectures for master-slave teleoperation, *IEEE Trans. on Control Systems Technology* **12**, 1, pp. 2–11.

[3] Anderson, R. J. and Spong, M. W. (1989). Bilateral control of teleoperators with time delay, *IEEE Trans. on Automatic Control* **34**, 5, pp. 494–501.

[4] Ang, W., Riviere, C. and Khosla, P. (2000). An active hand-held instrument for enhanced microsurgical accuracy, in *Medical Image Computing and Computer-Assisted Intervention* (Pittsburgh, PA).

[5] Arcara, P. and Melchiorri, C. (2002). Control schemes for teleoperation with time delay: A comparative study, *Robotics and Autonomous Systems* , 38, pp. 49–64.

[6] Arsenault, R. and Ware, C. (2000). Eye-hand co-ordination with force feedback, in *Proceedings of the SIGCHI conference on Human factors in computing systems* (The Hague, The Netherlands), pp. 408–414.

[7] Asari, V. K., Kumar, S. and Kassim, I. M. (2000). A fully autonomous microrobotic endoscopy system, *Journal of Intelligent and Robotic Systems* **28**, pp. 325–342.

[8] Ballantyne, G. H. (2002). Robotic surgery, telerobotic surgery, telepresence, and telementoring, *Surgical Endoscopy* **16**, 10, pp. 1389–1402.

[9] Berguer, R., Forkey, D. L. and Smith, W. D. (1999). Ergonomic problems associated with laparoscopic surgery, *Surg Endosc* **13**, 5, pp. 466 – 468.

[10] Berkelman, P., Whitcomb, L., Taylor, R. and Jensen, P. (2003). A miniature microsurgical instrument tip force sensor for enhanced force feedback during robot-assisted manipulation, *IEEE Transactions on Robotics and Automation* **19**, 5, pp. 917–922.

[11] Berkelmann, P. J., Rothbaum, D. L., Roy, J., III, S. L., Whitcomb, L. L., Hager, G., Jensen, P. S., Taylor, R. H. and Niparko, J. (2001). Performance evaluation of a cooperative manipulation microsurgical assistant robot applied to stapedotomy, in *Medical Image Computing and Computer-Assisted*

Interventions (Utrecht, The Netherlands), pp. 1426–1429.

[12] Bicchi, A., Canepa, G., Rossi, D. D., Iacconi, P. and Scillingo, E. P. (1996). A sensor-based minimally invasive surgery tool for detecting tissutal elastic properties, in *IEEE International Conference on Robotics and Automation*.

[13] Boerner, M. and Wiesel, U. (2001). European experience with an operative robot for primary and revision total hip – a summary of more than 3800 cases at bgu frankfurt, in *CAOS USA 2001* (Pittsburgh, PA).

[14] Breedveld, P., Stassen, H. G., Meijer, D. W. and Jakimowicz, J. J. (2000). Observation in laparoscopic surgery: overview of impeding effects and supporting aids, *Journal of Laparoendoscopic and Advanced Surgical Techniques* **10**, 5, pp. 231–241.

[15] Burdea, G. (1996). *Force and Touch Feedback for Virtual Reality* (John Wiley & Sons, New York).

[16] Butner, S. E. and Ghodoussi, M. (2003). Transforming a surgical robot for human telesurgery, *IEEE Transactions on Robotics and Automation* **19**, 5, pp. 818–824.

[17] Cabrera, J. B. D. and Narendra, K. S. (1999). Issues in the application of neural networks for tracking based on inverse control, *IEEE Transactions on Automatic Control* **44**, pp. 2007–27.

[18] Campion, G. and Hayward, V. (2005). Fundamental limits in the rendering of virtual haptic textures, in *Proceedings of First Joint Eurohaptics Conference and Symposium on Haptic Interfaces for Virtual Environments and Teleoperator Systems* (Pisa, Italy), pp. 263–270.

[19] Cavusoglu, M. C. and Feygin, D. (2002). A critical study of the mechanical and electrical properties of the PHANToM haptic interface and improvements for high performance control, *Presence: Teleoperators and Virtual Environments* **11**, 6, pp. 555–568.

[20] Cavusoglu, M. C., Williams, W., Tendick, F. and Sastry, S. (2003). Robotics for telesurgery: Second generation berkeley/ucsf laparoscopic telesurgical workstation and looking toward the future applications, *Industrial Robot* **30**, 1, pp. 22–29.

[21] Chang, S. O. and Okamura, A. M. (2004). Impedance-reflecting teleoperation with a real-time evolving neural network controller, in *Proceedings of IEEE/RSJ International Conference on Intelligent Robots and Systems*, pp. 2241–2246.

[22] Chen, E. and Marcus, B. (1998). Force feedback for surgical simulation, *Proceedings of the IEEE* **86**, 3, pp. 524–530.

[23] Cleary, K., Stoianovici, D., Glossop, N., Lindisch, D., Levy, E., Banovac, F., Stanimir, A. and Mazilu, D. (2001). Ct-directed robot biopsy testbed: Motivation and concept, in *SPIE Medical Imaging 2001 Conference* (San Diego, CA).

[24] Colgate, J. E. (1993). Robust impedance shaping telemanipulation, *IEEE Trans. on Robotics and Automation* **9**, 4, pp. 374–384.

[25] Dario, P., Carrozza, M. C., Marcacci, M., D'Attanasio, S., Magnami, B., Tonet, O. and Megali, G. (2000). A novel mechatronic tool for computer-assisted arthroscopy, *IEEE Transactions on Information Technology in*

Biomedicine **4**, 1, pp. 15–29.

[26] Dario, P., Hannaford, B. and Menciassi, A. (2003). Smart surgical tools and augmented devices, *IEEE Transactions on Robotics and Automation* **19**, 5, pp. 782–792.

[27] Davies, B. L. (2002). Robotic surgery: at the cutting edge of technology, in *Proceedings of 7th International Workshop on Advanced Motion Control*, pp. 15–18.

[28] de Wit, C. C., Olsson, H., Astrom, K. J. and Lischinsky, P. (1995). A new model for control of systems with friction, *IEEE Transactions on Automatic Control* **40**, 3, pp. 419–425.

[29] Debus, T., Jang, T.-J., Dupont, P. and Howe, R. (2004). Multi-channel vibrotactile display for teleoperated assembly, *International Journal of Control, Automation, and Systems* **2**, 3, pp. 390–397.

[30] et al., M. C. C. (Aug 1999). A laparoscopic telesurgical workstation, *IEEE Transactions on Robotics and Automation* **15**, pp. 728–739.

[31] Faraz, A. and Payandeh, S. (1997a). A robotics case study: Optimal design for laparoscopic positioning stands, in *IEEE International Conference on Robotics and Automation*, Vol. 2.

[32] Faraz, A. and Payandeh, S. (1997b). Synthesis and workspace study of endoscopic extenders with flexible stem, *Journal of Mechanical Design* **119**, 3, pp. 801–808.

[33] Faraz, A., Payandeh, S. and Nagy, A. (1995). Issues and design concepts in endoscopic extenders, in *IFAC Man/Machine Systems* (Boston).

[34] Feygin, D., Keehner, M. and Tendick, F. (2002). Haptic guidance: Experimental evaluation of a haptic training method for a perceptual motor skill, in *Proceedings of the 10th Symposium on Haptic Interfaces for Virtual Environment and Teleoperator Systems* (Orlando, Florida), pp. 40–47.

[35] Fite, K. B., Shao, L. and Goldfarb, M. (2004). Loop shaping for transparency and stability robustness in bilateral telemanipulation, *IEEE Transactions on Robotics and Automation* **20**, 3, pp. 620–624.

[36] Fitts, P. M. and Peterson, J. (1964). Information capacity of discrete motor responses, *Journal of Experimental Psychology* **67**, 2, pp. 103–112.

[37] Fukuda, T., Guo, S., Kosuge, K., Arai, F., Negoro, M. and Nakabayashi, K. (1994). Micro active catheter system with multi degrees of freedom, in *IEEE International Conference on Robotics and Automation* (San Diego, California).

[38] Fukuda, T. and Shibata, T. (1992). Theory and application of neural networks for industrial control systems, *IEEE Transactions on Industrial Electronics* **39**, pp. 472–89.

[39] Furukawa, T., Morikawa, Y., Ozawa, S., Wakabayashi, G. and Kitajima, M. (2001). The revolution of computer-aided surgery – the dawn of robotic surgery, *Minimally Invasive Therapy & Allied Technologies* **10**, 6, pp. 283–288.

[40] Gao, F. and Gruver, W. A. (1997). Performance evaluation criteria for analysis and design of robotic mechanisms, in *The 8th International Conference on Advanced Robotics* (Monterey, CA).

[41] Gerovichev, O., Marayong, P. and Okamura, A. (2002). The effect of visual and haptic feedback on manual and teleoperated needle insertion, in T. Dohi and R. Kikinis (eds.), *Proceedings of the Fifth International Conference on Medical Image Computing and Computer Assisted Intervention – Lecture Notes in Computer Science (Vol. 2488)*, pp. 147–154.

[42] Glauser, D., Clavel, R., Baumann, R. and Maeder, W. (1997). The pantoscope: A spherical remote-center-of-motion parallel manipulator for force reflection, in *IEEE International Conference on Robotics and Automation* (Albuquerque, NM).

[43] Gomes, M. P. S. F., Barrett, A. R. W. and Davies, B. L. (2001). Computer-assisted soft-tissue surgery training and monitoring, in *International Conference on Medical Image Computing and Computer-Assisted Intervention*, Vol. 2.

[44] Gosselin, C. and Angeles, J. (1991). A global performance index for the kinematic optimization of robotic manipulators, *Transactions of the ASME, Journal of Mechanical Design* **113**, pp. 220–226.

[45] Gray, B. L. and Fearing, R. S. (1996). A surface micromachined microtactile sensor array, in *IEEE International Conference on Robotics and Automation*, Vol. 1 (Minneapolis, Minnesota).

[46] Gupta, R., Sheridan, T. and Whitney, D. (1997). Experiments using multimodal virtual environments in design for assembly analysis, *Presence: Teleoperators and Virtual Environments* **6**, 3, pp. 318–338.

[47] Haga, Y., Tanahasi, Y. and Esashi, M. (1998). Small diameter active catheter using shape memory alloy, in *IEEE MEMS Workshop* (Heidelberig).

[48] Hannaford, B. (1989). A design framework for teleoperators with kinesthetic feedback, *IEEE Transactions on Robotics and Automation* **5**, pp. 426–434.

[49] Hannaford, B. and Wood, L. (1989). Performance evaluation of a 6 axis high fidelity generalized force reflecting teleoperator, in *Proceedings of JPL/NASA Conference on Space Telerobotics* (Pasadena, CA), pp. 89–97.

[50] Harris, S., Arambula-Cosio, F., Mei, Q., Hibberd, R. D., Davies, B. L., Wickham, J. E., Nathan, M. and Kundu, B. (1997). The probot - an active robot for prostate resection, *Journal of Engineering in Medicine, Proc Inst Mech Eng, Part H.* **211**, 4, pp. 317–325.

[51] Hashizume, M., Shimada, M., Tomikawa, M., Ikeda, Y., Takahashi, I., Abe, R., Koga, F., Gotoh, N., Konishi, K., Maehara, S. and Sugimachi, K. (2002). Early experiences of endoscopic procedures in general surgery assisted by a computer-enhanced surgical system, *Surg Endosc* **16**, 8, pp. 1187–1191.

[52] Hashtrudi-Zaad, K. and Salcudean, S. E. (2002). Transparency in time delay systems and the effect of local force feedback for transparent teleoperation, *IEEE Transactions on Robotics and Automation* **18**, 1, pp. 108–114.

[53] Haykin, S. (1970). *Active Network Theory* (Addison-Wesley, Reading, MA).

[54] Hayward, V. (2001). Survey of haptic interface research at mcgill university, in *Workshop on "Advances in Interactive Multimodal Telepresence Sys-*

tems" (Munich, Germany).

[55] Hayward, V., Astley, O. R., Cruz-Hernandez, M., Grant, D. and Robles-De-La-Torre, G. (2004). Haptic interfaces and devices, *Sensor Review* **24**, 1, pp. 16–29.

[56] Hayward, V., Gregorio, P., Astley, O., Greenish, S. and Doyon, M. (1998). Freedom-7: A high fidelity seven axis haptic device with application to surgical training, Experimental Robotics, Lecture Notes in Control and Information Science 232, Springer Verlag.

[57] Hokayem, P. F. and Spong, M. W. (2006). Bilateral teleoperation: An historical survey, *Automatica* **42**, 12, pp. 2035–2057.

[58] Holden, J. G., Flach, J. M. and Donchin, Y. (1999). Perceptual-motor coordination in an endoscopic surgery simulation, *Surg Endosc* **13**, 2, pp. 127–132.

[59] Howe, R. and Matsuoka, Y. (1999). Robotics for surgery, *Annu. Rev. Biomed. Eng.* **01**, pp. 211–240.

[60] Howe, R., Peine, W. J., Kantarinis, D. A. and Son, J. S. (1995). Remote palpation technology, *IEEE Engineering in Medicine and Biology Magazine* **14**, 3, pp. 318–323.

[61] Hurmuzlu, Y., Ephanov, A. and Stoianovici, D. (1998). Effect of a pneumatically driven haptic interface on the perceptional capabilities of human operators, *Presence: Teleoperators and Virtual Environments* **7**, 3, pp. 290–307.

[62] Ikuta, K., Tsukamot, M. and Hirose, S. (1998). Shape memory alloy servo actuator system with electric resistence feedback and application for active endoscope, in *IEEE International Conference on Robotics and Automation* (Leven, Belgium).

[63] Ikuta, K., Yamamoto, K. and Sasaki, K. (2003). Development of remote microsurgery robot and new surgical procedure for deep and narrow space, in *IEEE International Conference on Robotics and Automation* (Taipei, Taiwan), pp. 1103–1108.

[64] Imaida, T., Yokokohji, Y., Doi, T., Oda, M. and Yoshikawa, T. (2004). Ground-space bilateral teleoperation of ETS-VII robot arm by direct bilateral coupling under 7-s time delay condition, *IEEE Transactions on Robotics and Automation* **20**, 3, pp. 499–511.

[65] Integrated Surgical Systems Inc. (2007). *http://www.robodoc.com/eng/neuromate.html.*

[66] Jakopec, M., Baena, F. R., Harris, S. J., Gomes, P., Cohh., J. and Davies, B. L. (2003). The hands-on orthopaedic robot "acrobot": early clinical trials of total knee replacement surgery, *IEEE Transactions on Robotics and Automation* **19**, 5, pp. 902–911.

[67] Jakopec, M., Harris, S. J., Baena, F. R. Y., Gomes, P., Cobb, J. and Davies, B. L. (2001). The first clinical application of a hands-on robotic knee surgery system, *Computer Aided Surgery* **6**, pp. 329–339.

[68] Joice, P., Hanna, G. B. and Cuschieri, A. (1998). Errors enacted during endoscopic surgery – a human reliability analysis, *Applied Ergonomics* **29**, 6, pp. 409–414.

[69] Kang, H. and Wen, J. T. (2001). Robotic assistants aid surgeons during minimally invasive procedures, *IEEE Engineering in Medicine and Biology* , pp. 94–104.

[70] Kattavenos, N., Lawrenson, B., Frank, T., Pridham, M., Keatch, R. and Cuschieri, A. (2004). Force-sensitive tactile sensor for minimal access surgery, *Minimally Invasive Therapy & Allied Technologies* **13**, 1, pp. 42–46.

[71] Kavoussi, L. R., Moore, R. G., b. Adams, J. and Partin, A. W. (1995). Comparison of robotic versus human laparoscopic camera control, *J Urol* **154**, pp. 2134–2146.

[72] Kazerooni, H. (1990). Human-robot interaction via the transfer of power and information signals, *IEEE Transactions on Systems, Man and Cybernetics* **20**, 2, pp. 450–463.

[73] Kermani, M. R., Patel, R. V. and Moallem, M. (2005). Case studies of friction identifcation in robotic manipulators, in *Proceedings of IEEE International Conference on Control Applications* (Toronto, Canada).

[74] Kitagawa, M., Dokko, D., Okamura, A. M. and Yuh, D. D. (2005). Effect of sensory substitution on suture manipulation forces for robotic surgical systems, *Journal of Thoracic and Cardiovascular Surgery* **129**, 1, pp. 151–158.

[75] Kornbluh, R., Pelrine, R., Eckerle, J. and Joseph, J. (1998). Electrostrictive polymer artificial muscle actuators, in *IEEE International Conference on Robotics and Automation* (Leuven, Belgium).

[76] Kumar, R., Barnes, A., Hager, G., Jensen, P. and Taylor, R. (2001). Application of task-level augmentation for cooperative fine manipulation tasks in surgery, in *Medical Image Computing and Computer-Assisted Intervention* (Utrecht, The Netherlands).

[77] Kwon, D. S., Lee, J. J., Yoon, Y. S., Ko, S. Y., Kim, J., Chung, J. H., Won, C. H. and Kim, J. H. (2002). The mechanism and the registration method of a surgical robot for hip arthroplasty, in *IEEE International Conference on Robotics and Automation*.

[78] Kypson, A. P., Nifong, L. W. and Chitwood, W. R. (2003). Robotic cardiac surgery, *Journal of Long-Term Effects of Medical Implants* **13**, 6, pp. 451–464.

[79] Lawrence, D. A. (1993). Stability and transparency in bilateral teleoperation, *IEEE Transactions on Robotics & Automation* **9**, pp. 624–637.

[80] Lazeroms, M. (1999). *Force Reflection for Telemanipulation Applied to Minimally Invasive Surgery*, Ph.D. thesis, Delft University of Technology.

[81] Louw, D. F., Fielding, T., McBeth, P. B., Gregoris, D., Newhook, P. and Sutherland, G. R. (2004). Surgical robotics: a review and neurosurgical prototype development, *Neurosurgery* **54**, 3, pp. 525–537.

[82] Love, L. and Book, W. (2004). Force reflecting teleoperation with adaptive impedance control, *IEEE Transactions on Systems, Man and Cybernetics – Part B* **34**, 1, pp. 159–165.

[83] Lueth, T. and Beir, J. (1999). Robot assisted intevention in surgery, in *Neuronavigation – Neurosurgical and Computer Scientific Aspects* (Springer

Verlag).

[84] Lum, M. J., Rosen, J., Sinanan, M. N. and Hannaford, B. (2004). Kinematic optimization of a spherical mechanism for a minimally invasive surgical robot, in *Proceedings of IEEE International Conference on Robotics and Automation* (New Orleans, LA), pp. 829–834.

[85] Madhani, A., Niemeyer, G. and Jr., K. S. (1998). The black falcon – a tele-operated surgical instrument for minimally invasive surgery, in *IEEE/RSJ International Conference on Intelligent Robots and Systems* (Victoria, BC, Canada).

[86] Malpass, L. (1963). *Motor skills in mental deficiency. Handbook of Mental Deficiency* (McGraw-Hill, New York).

[87] Mason, A., Walji, M., Lee, E. and MacKenzie, C. (2001). Reaching movements to augmented and graphic objects in virtual environments, in *Proceedings of the SIGCHI conference on Human factors in computing systems* (Seattle, Washington), pp. 426–433.

[88] Massie, T. (1993). *Design of a Three Degree of Freedom Force-Reflecting Haptic Interface*, B.S. thesis, MIT.

[89] Massimino, M. (1992). *Sensory substitution for force feedback in teleoperation*, Ph.D. thesis, MIT.

[90] Matsuhira, N., Jinno, M., Miyagawa, T., Sunaoshi, T., Hato, T., Morikawa, Y., Furukawa, T., Ozawa, S., Kitajima, M. and Nakazawa, K. (2003). Development of a functional model for a master-slave combined manipulator for laparoscopic surgery, *Advanced Robotics* **17**, 6, pp. 523–539.

[91] McColl, R., Brown, I., Seligman, C., Lim, F. and Alsaraira, A. (2006). Haptic rendering and perception studies for laparoscopic surgery simulation. in *Proceedings of the 28th IEEE Engineering in Medicine and Biology Conference* (New York, NY), pp. 833–836.

[92] Mitsuishi, M., Warisawa, S. I., Tsuda, T., Higuchi, T., Koizumi, N., Hashizume, H. and Fujiwara, K. (2001). Remote ultrasound diagnostic system, in *IEEE International Conference on Robotics and Automation* (Seoul, Korea).

[93] Mitsuishi, M., Watanabe, T., Nakanishi, H., Hori, T., Watanabe, H. and Kramer, B. (1995). A telemicrosurgery system with colocated view and operation points and rotational-force-feedback-free master manipulator, in *International Symposium on Medical Robotics and Computer-Assisted Surgery* (Baltimore, MD).

[94] Moody, L., Baber, C., Arvanitis, T. N. and Elliott, M. (2003). Objective metrics for the evaluation of simple surgical skills in real and virtual domains, *Presence: Teleoperators & Virtual Environments* **12**, 2, pp. 207–221.

[95] Morimoto, A. K., Floral, R. D., Kuhlman, J. L., Zucker, K. A., Couret, M. J., Bocklage, T., MacFarlane, T. I. and Kory, L. (1997). Force sensor for laparoscopic babcock, in K. S. M. et al. (ed.), *Medicine Meets Virtual Reality*, Vol. 2 (Washington DC).

[96] Munir, S. and Book, W. J. (2002). Internet-based teleoperation using wave variables with prediction, *IEEE/ASME Trans. on Mechatronics* **7**, 2, pp. 124–133.

[97] Narumiya, H. (1993). Micromachine technology (intraluminal diagnostic & therapeutic system), in *Workshop on Micromachine Technologies and Systems* (Tokyo, Japan).

[98] Negoro, M., Takahashi, I., Nakabayashi, K., Fukui, K. and Sugita, K. (1994). Current situation of intravascular neurosurgery and its future, in *The 5th International Symposium on Micro Machine and Human Science* (Nagoya, Japan).

[99] Ng, W. S., Phee, S. J. and Seow-Choen, F. (2000). Robotic endoscope and an autonomous pipe robot for performing endoscopic procedures, U.s. patent 6,162,171.

[100] Nicosia, S. and Tomei, P. (1990). Robot control by using only joint position measurements, *IEEE Transactions on Automatic Control* **35**, 9, pp. 1058–1061.

[101] Niemeyer, G. and Slotine, J. J. E. (1991). Stable adaptive teleoperation, *IEEE Journal of Oceanic Eng.* **16**, 1, pp. 152–162.

[102] Niemeyer, G. and Slotine, J. J. E. (2004). Telemanipulation with time delays, *Int. Journal of Robotic Research* **23**, 9, pp. 873–890.

[103] Nishikawa, A., Hosoi, T., Koara, K., Negoro, D., Hikita, A., Asano, S., Kakutani, H., Miyazaki, F., Sekimoto, M., Yasui, M., Miyake, Y., Takiguchi, S. and Monden, M. (2003). FAce MOUSe: A novel human-machine interface for controlling the position of a laparoscope, *IEEE Transactions on Robotics and Automation* **19**, 5, pp. 825–841.

[104] Okamura, A. M., Simone, C. and O'Leary, M. D. (2004). Force modeling for needle insertion into soft tissue, *IEEE Transactions on Biomedical Engineering* **51**, 10, pp. 1707–1716.

[105] Omote, K., Feussner, H., Ungeheuer, A., Arbter, K., Wei, G. Q., Siewert, J. R. and Hirzinger, G. (1999). Self-guided robotic camera control for laparoscopic surgery compared with human camera control, *Am J Surg* **177**, pp. 321–324.

[106] Ortmaier, T., Reintsema, D., Seibold, U., Hagn, U. and Hirzinger, G. (2001). The DLR minimally invasive robotics surgery scenario, Workshop on Advances in Interactive Multimodal Telepresence Systems, Munich, Germany.

[107] Ottensmeyer, M. (1996). *Telerobotic Surgery – Feedback Time Delay Effects on Task Assignment*, Master's thesis, MIT, Cambridge, MA.

[108] Ottensmeyer, M. P. and Salisbury, J. K. (2001). In vivo data acquisition instrument for solid organ mechanical property measurement, in *Medical Image Computing and Computer-Assisted Intervention*.

[109] Peirs, J., Reynaerts, D., and Brussel, H. V. (2000). Design of miniature parallel manipulators for integration in a self-propelling endoscope, *Sensors and Actuators* **85**, pp. 409–417.

[110] Phee, L., Accoto, D., Menciassi, A., Stefanini, C., Carrozza, M. C. and Dario, P. (2002a). Analysis and development of locomotion devices for the gastrointestinal tract, *IEEE Transactions on Biomedical Engineering* **49**, pp. 613–616.

[111] Phee, L., Menciassi, A., Gorini, S., Pernorio, G., Arena, A. and Dario, P.

(2002b). An innovative locomotion principle for minirobots moving in the gastrointestinal tract, in *IEEE International Conference on Robotics and Automation* (Washington DC).

[112] Polushin, I., Liu, P. and Lung, C.-H. (2006). A control scheme for stable force-reflecting teleoperation over ip networks, *IEEE Transactions on Systems, Man and Cybernetics - Part B* **36**, 4, pp. 930–939.

[113] Richards, C., Rosen, J., Hannaford, B., Pellegrini, C. and Sinanan, M. (2000). Skills evaluation in minimally invasive surgery using force/torque signatures, *Surg Endosc* **14**, pp. 791–798.

[114] Rosen, J., Brown, J. D., Chang, L., Barreca, M., Sinanan, M. and Hannaford, B. (2002). The bluedragon – a system for measuring the kinematics and dynamics of minimally invasive surgical tools in-vivo, in *IEEE International Conference on Robotics and Automation*, Vol. 2, pp. 1876–1881.

[115] Rosen, J., Hannaford, B., MacFarlane, M. and Sinanan, M. (1999). Force controlled and teleoperated endoscopic grasper for minimally invasive surgery - experimental performance evaluation, *IEEE Transactions on Biomedical Engineering* **46**, pp. 1212–1221.

[116] Rothbaum, D. L., Roy, J., Berkelman, P., Hager, G., Stoianovici, D., Taylor, R. H., Whitcomb, L. L., Francis, M. H. and Niparko, J. K. (2002). Robot-assisted stapedotomy: micropick fenestration of the stapes footplate, *Otolaryngology – Head and Neck Surgery* **127**, pp. 417–426.

[117] Ruurda, J. P., Broeders, I. A., Pulles, B., Kappelhof, F. M. and van der Werken, C. (2004). Manual robot assisted endoscopic suturing: time-action analysis in an experimental model, *Surgical Endoscopy* **18**, 8, pp. 1249–1252.

[118] Santa, A. D., Mazzoldi, A. and Rossi, D. D. (1996). Steerable microcatheters actuated by embedded conducting polymer structures, *Journal of Intelligence Material Systems and Structures* **7**, pp. 292–300.

[119] Schneider, O., Troccaz, J., Chavanon, O. and Blin, D. (2000). Padyc: a synergistic robot for cardiac puncturing, in *IEEE International Conference on Robotics and Automation*.

[120] Sheridan, T. B. (1993). Space teleoperation through time delay: Review and prognosis, *IEEE Trans. on Robotics* **9**, 5, pp. 592–606.

[121] Sherman, A., Cavusoglu, M. and Tendick, F. (2000). Comparison of teleoperator control architectures for palpation task, in S. S. Nair (ed.), *Proc. ASME Dynamic Systems and Control Division*, Vol. DSC 69-2, pp. 1261–8.

[122] Shimoga, K. (1993). A survey of perceptual feedback issues in dextrous telemanipulation: Part I. Finger Force Feedback, in *Proc. IEEE Annual Virtual Reality Int. Symp* (Seattle, Washington), pp. 263–270.

[123] Slatkin, A. B., Burdick, J. and Grundfest, W. (1995). The development of a robotic endoscope, in *IEEE/RSJ International Conference on Intelligent Robots and Systems*, Vol. 2, pp. 162–171.

[124] Soderstrom, T. and Stoica, P. (1989). *System Identification* (Prentice Hall International Ltd).

[125] Starkie, S. J. and Davies, B. L. (2001). Advances in active constraints and their application to minimally invasive surgery, in *Proceedings of the*

4th International Conference on Medical Image Computing and Computer-Assisted Intervention.

[126] Stephenson, E. J., Sankholkar, S., Ducko, C. T. and Damiano, R. J. J. (1998). Robotically assisted microsurgery for endoscopic coronary artery bypass grafting, *The Annals of Thoracic Surgery* **66**, 3, pp. 1064–1067.

[127] Sturges, R. and Laowattana, S. (1991). A flexible, tendon-controlled device for endoscopy, in *IEEE International Conference on Robotics and Automation* (Sacramento, California).

[128] Su, L. M., Stoianovici, D., Jarrett, T. W. and et al., A. P. (2002). Robotic percutaneous access to the kidney: comparison with standard manual access, *Journal of Endourology* **16**, pp. 471–475.

[129] Sung, G. T. and Gill, I. S. (2001). Robotic laparoscopic surgery: a comparison of the da Vinci and Zeus systems, *Urology* **58**, 6, pp. 893–898.

[130] Suzumori, K., Iikura, S. and Tanaka, H. (1991). Development of flexible microactuator and its applications to robotics mechanisms, in *IEEE International Conference on Robotics and Automation* (Sacramento, California).

[131] Taffinder, N., Sutton, C., Fishwick, R. J., McManus, I. C. and Darzi, A. (1998). Validation of virtual reality to teach and assess psychomotor skills in laparoscopic surgery: Results from randomised controlled studies using the MIST VR laparoscopic simulator, in *Proceedings of Medicine Meets Virtual Reality*, pp. 124–130.

[132] Tahmasebi, A. M., Taati, B., Mobasser, F. and Hashtrudi-Zaad, K. (2005). Dynamic parameter identification and analysis of a PHANToM haptic device, in *Proceedings of the 2005 IEEE Conference on Control Applications*, pp. 1251–1256.

[133] Tanner, N. A. and Niemeyer, G. (2006). High-frequency acceleration feedback in wave variable telerobotics, *IEEE/ASME Trans. on Mechatronics* **11**, 2, pp. 119–127.

[134] Taylor, R., Jensen, P., Whitcomb, L., Barnes, A., Kumar, R., Stoianovici, D., Gupta, P., Wang, Z. X., deJuan, E. and Kavoussi, L. (1999). Steady-hand robotic system for microsurgical augmentation, *International Journal of Robotics Research* **18**, pp. 1201–1210.

[135] Taylor, R. and Stoianovici, D. (2003). Medical robotics in computer-integrated surgery, *IEEE Transactions on Robotics and Automation* **19**, pp. 765–781.

[136] Taylor, R. H., Funda, J., Eldridge, B., Gruben, K., LaRose, D., Gomory, S., Talamini, M., Kavoussi, L. and Anderson, J. (1995). A telerobotic assistant for laparoscopic surgery, *IEEE Eng. Med. Biol. Mag.* , pp. 279–291.

[137] Taylor, R. H., Paul, H. A., Kazandzides, P., Mittelstadt, B. D., Hanson, W., Zuhars, J. F., Williamson, B., Musits, B. L., Glassman, E. and Bargar, W. L. (1994). An image-directed robotic system for precise orthopaedic surgery, *IEEE Transactions on Robotics and Automation* **10**, pp. 261–275.

[138] Taylor II, R., Hudson, T., Seeger, A., Weber, H., Juliano, J. and Helser, A. (2001). VRPN: A device-independent, network-transparent VR peripheral system, in *Proceedings of ACM Symposium on Virtual Reality Software & Technology* (Baniff, Alberta, Canada), pp. 55–61.

[139] Tendick, F., Jennings, R., Tharp, G. and Stark, L. (1993). Sensing and manipulation problems in endoscopic surgery: Experiment, analysis and observation, *Presence: Teleoperators and Virtual Environments* **2**, 1, pp. 66–81.

[140] Tendick, F., Jennings, R., Tharp, G. and Stark, L. (1996). *Perception and manipulation problems in endoscopic surgery. In: Computer-Integrated Surgery: Technology and Clinical Applications* (MIT Press, Cambridge, Massachusetts).

[141] Tendick, F., Sastry, S. S., Fearing, R. S. and Cohn, M. (1998). Applications of micromechatronics in minimally invasive surgery, *IEEE/ASME Transactions on Mechatronics* **3**, 1, pp. 34–42.

[142] Tholey, G. and Desai, J. (2004). On-site three dimensional force sensing capability in a laparoscopic grasper, *Industrial Robot: An International Journal* **31**, 6, pp. 509–518.

[143] Treat, M. R. and Trimmer, W. S. (1997). Self-propelled endoscope using pressure driven linear actuators, U.s. patent 5,595,565.

[144] Trejos, A., Salcudean, S., Sassani, F. and Lichtenstein, S. (1999). On the feasibility of a moving support for surgery on the beating heart, in *Medical Image Computing and Computer-Assisted Interventions* (Cambridge, U.K.).

[145] Verner, L. N. and Okamura, A. M. (2006). Sensor/actuator asymmetries in telemanipulators: Implications of partial force feedback, in *Proceedings of the 14th Symposium on Haptic Interfaces for Virtual Environments and Teleoperator Systems* (New York, NY), pp. 309–314.

[146] Vlachos, K., Papadopoulos, E. and Mitropoulos, D. (2003). Design and implementation of a haptic device for training in urological operations, *IEEE Transactions on Robotics and Automation* **19**, pp. 801–808.

[147] Wagner, C., Stylopoulos, N. and Howe, R. (2002). The role of force feedback in surgery: Analysis of blunt dissection, in *10th Symp. on Haptic Interfaces for Virtual Environment and Teleoperator Systems* (Orlando), pp. 68–74.

[148] Wang, X.-G., Moallem, M. and Patel, R. V. (2003). An internet-based distributed multiple-telerobot system, *IEEE Transactions on Systems, Man and Cybernetics - Part A* **33**, 5, pp. 627–633.

[149] Wiesel, U., Lahmer, A., Tenbusch, M. and Borner, M. (2001). Total knee replacement using the robodoc system, in *First Annual. Meeting of CAOS International* (Davos, Switzerland).

[150] Woo, K. Y., Jin, B. D. and Kwon, D. (1998). A 6dof force reflecting hand controller using the five-bar parallel mechanism, in *IEEE International Conference on Robotics and Automation* (Leuven, Belgium).

[151] Wu, D., Hou, Y. T., Zhu, W., Zhang, Y. Q. and Peha, J. M. (2001). Streaming video over internet: approaches and directions, *IEEE Transactions on Circuits and Systems for Video Technology* **11**, pp. 282–300.

[152] Yamamoto, S. and Kimura, H. (1995). On structured singular values of reciprocal matrices, *Proc. of the American Control Conference* , pp. 3358–3359.

[153] Yokokohji, Y. and Yoshikawa, T. (1994). Bilateral control of master-slave

manipulators for ideal kinesthetic coupling–formulation and experiment, *IEEE Transactions on Robotics and Automation* **10**, 5, pp. 605–620.

[154] Zhang, X. and Payandeh, S. (2002). Application of visual tracking for robotic-assisted laparoscopic surgery, *Journal of Robotics Systems* **19**, 7, pp. 315–328.

Index